The Johns Hopkins Atlas of Human Functional Anatomy

Original Illustrations, with Descriptive Legends, by
Leon Schlossberg

Text Edited by **George D. Zuidema, M.D.**

Third Edition
Revised and
Expanded

The Johns Hopkins Atlas of

Human Functional Anatomy

The Johns Hopkins University Press · Baltimore and London

To Jean and Joan

Plates 3, 4, and 5, courtesy of the Medical Models Laboratory;
plates 11, 12, 13, 18, 26, 44, 45, 46, 47, 48, 49, 50, 51, 52, 53, 54,
55, 56, 57, 58, 60, 61, and 62 all originally published by W. B.
Saunders Company; plates 14 and 15, courtesy of the Medical
Department, U.S. Navy; plates 2, 21, 31, and 37, courtesy of
Winthrop Laboratories. Plate 43 first appeared in *Atlas of Nuclear
Medicine,* vol. 2, by Frank H. Deland and Henry N. Wagner (Phila-
delphia: W. B. Saunders Company, 1970). All are reproduced with
permission.

Printed in the United States of America

The Johns Hopkins University Press, 701 West 40th Street,
Baltimore, Maryland 21211
The Johns Hopkins Press Ltd., London

Originally published, 1977
Second edition, 1980
Third edition, 1986

Library of Congress Cataloging in Publication Data

Main entry under title:
The Johns Hopkins atlas of human functional anatomy.

   Includes index.
   1. Anatomy, Human. 2. Anatomy, Human—Atlases.
I. Schlossberg, Leon. II. Zuidema, George D.
III. Johns Hopkins University. School of Medicine.
[DNLM: 1. Anatomy—atlases. 2. Physiology—atlases. QS 17 J64]
QM23.2.J63 1986   611   85-22031
ISBN 0-8018-3282-9
ISBN 0-8018-3283-7 (pbk.)

Contributors

The Johns Hopkins University School of Medicine

FACULTY

William R. Bell, M.D. Professor of Medicine and Professor of Radiology

Robert K. Brawley, M.D. Associate Professor of Surgery

Rainer M. E. Engel, M.D. Associate Professor of Urology

Melvin H. Epstein, M.D. Associate Professor of Neurological Surgery and Assistant Professor of Emergency Medicine

Margaret M. Fletcher, M.D. Assistant Professor of Otolaryngology/Head and Neck Surgery

Vincent L. Gott, M.D. Richard Bennett Darnall Professor of Surgery

David W. Heese, D.D.S. Assistant Professor of Dental Surgery

Thomas R. Hendrix, M.D. Professor of Medicine, Paulson Professor of Gastroenterology, and Chief of Gastroenterology

Charles E. Iliff, M.D. Professor Emeritus of Ophthalmology

Donlin M. Long, M.D., Ph.D. Professor of Neurological Surgery and Chairman of the Department of Neurological Surgery

George T. Nager, M.D. Andelot Professor Emeritus of Otolaryngology/Head and Neck Surgery

James J. Ryan, M.D. Assistant Professor of Plastic Surgery

Leon Schlossberg Assistant Professor of Art as Applied to Medicine

Vernon T. Tolo, M.D. Associate Professor of Orthopaedic Surgery and Chief of Pediatric Orthopaedic Surgery

George B. Udvarhelyi, M.D. Professor Emeritus of Neurological Surgery and Associate Professor Emeritus of Radiology

Henry N. Wagner, Jr., M.D. Professor and Director of the Division of Nuclear Medicine and Radiation Health

FORMER FACULTY

Donald S. Gann, M.D. J. Murray Beardsley Professor of Surgery and Chairman of the Department of Surgery, Brown University, and Surgeon-in-Chief, Department of Surgery, Rhode Island Hospital, Providence, Rhode Island

James L. Hughes, M.D. Professor of Orthopaedic Surgery and Chief of the Division of Orthopaedic Surgery, University of Mississippi Medical Center, Jackson, Mississippi

James P. Isaacs, M.D. Active Staff, Nanticoke Memorial Hospital, Seaford, Delaware

Howard W. Jones, Jr., M.D. Professor of Obstetrics and Gynecology, Eastern Virginia Medical School, Norfolk, Virginia, and Professor Emeritus, The Johns Hopkins University School of Medicine

H. Lorrin Lau, M.D. Associate Professor, University of Hawaii School of Medicine, Honolulu, Hawaii

John J. White, M.D. Director, Division of Pediatric Surgery and Professor of Surgery and Pediatrics, Albany Medical College of Union University, Albany, New York

George D. Zuidema, M.D. Vice Provost for Medical Affairs and Professor of Surgery, The University of Michigan, Ann Arbor, Michigan

Contents

PLATES

Preface to the Third Edition

This volume unites the unique artistic talents of Leon Schlossberg with a text written by the faculty of The Johns Hopkins University School of Medicine. The book itself is designed to present basic anatomy to students of medicine and the allied health professions as well as to undergraduates, and does so in a manner that emphasizes function as well as structure. The text covers basic principles, with sufficient attention to detail to permit students to orient themselves to the subject and obtain a working knowledge of anatomical systems and specialized organs. The functional approach is of help in understanding interrelationships. New plates, which illustrate additional material on embryology and the cranium and autonomic nervous system, the liver and esophagus, the intestines, hernia, and the perineum, have been added, together with expanded text on these areas. The result is an improved, more extensive volume, which should serve as a useful handbook and a departure point for the detailed study of anatomy, where necessary, by other techniques. In certain instances, newer anatomical nomenclature differs from that generally used by clinicians. Where this situation occurs, we have elected to use the terms that are used most widely by physicians and surgeons in clinical practice, for it is this terminology the student is also most likely to use. The artist and the authors believe that this book will be a useful introduction to this phase of health science education.

George D. Zuidema, M.D.

Acknowledgments

I am indebted to Dr. George D. Zuidema for his interest in the idea for this book and for his help in bringing it to fruition. To the physicians and surgeons in many of the specialties at The Johns Hopkins University School of Medicine go most sincere thanks for the text they contributed and for the untiring manner in which they cooperated in consultations and in offering their criticisms. It is a distinct privilege for a medical illustrator to have access to the authoritative advice of anatomical, medical, and surgical experts. I owe a personal debt to the late Max Broedel, founder of the Department of Art as Applied to Medicine, for it was he who almost single-handedly created at the Hopkins Medical Institutions a niche for medical illustration, from which has developed an excellent professional relationship between physician and illustrator.

I would like to thank the Medical Department of Winthrop Laboratories for their generous permission to use several of the illustrations that were originally produced for them. The W. B. Saunders Company kindly allowed me to reuse a number of my plates from the Schlossberg-Zuidema *Atlas of Surgical Anatomy of the Abdomen and Pelvis* and one of my illustrations from Deland and Wagner's *Atlas of Nuclear Medicine*. To the Medical Department of the U.S. Navy I extend grateful acknowledgment for the use of the plates on blood I created for them, and to the Medical Models Laboratory I offer thanks for allowing me to reproduce here the comprehensive portrayal of the skeletal anatomy that they originally commissioned from me.

To my wife, Jean, who encouraged me from the outset of this project, I am especially grateful. She skillfully translated my notes into understandable labels, with which she personally prepared the initial overlays for the illustrations.

To Mrs. Diane Cyryca and Ms. Nona Mustard, of the administrative secretarial staff of the Department of Surgery at the Hopkins School of Medicine and the office of the vice provost for medical affairs of the University of Michigan, I extend sincere appreciation from myself as well as on behalf of my colleague Dr. Zuidema.

Leon Schlossberg

Introduction

Dorland's *Medical Dictionary* defines anatomy as: "1. The science of the structure of the animal body and the relation of its parts. It is largely based on dissection, from which it obtains its name. 2. Dissection of an organized body." The definition continues to include applied anatomy, as well as artificial, artistic, microscopic, classic, comparative, general, gross, biological, medical, pathological, physiological, and other subdivisions of the study of anatomy. Physiology is defined in Dorland's as: "The science which treats of the functions of the living organism and its parts." It is this area—functional living anatomy and the component structures of the body and the relation of its parts—that this work will endeavor to depict.

The key illustration in the chapter on the central nervous system is entitled "The Five Senses of Consciousness": hearing, seeing, tasting, smelling, and sense of movement and position of the body. These faculties are defined in accompanying legends and are further elucidated in the text describing the anatomy and functions of the brain, nerves, and spinal cord. Other body functions treated in like manner include skeletal, articulatory, muscular, alimentary, respiratory, urinary, reproductive, lymphatic, endocrine, integumentary, and autonomic and somatic nerve functions, and blood and cerebrospinal fluid circulation. The activity of these systems represents total body function. The organs—their structure and their topographical relationships—are illustrated and defined by the captions and accompanying descriptive text. Concerted efforts have been made to present the anatomy and function to facilitate the understanding of clinical conditions and diagnostic and corrective procedures. Since living anatomy and function are depicted, some of the study and reference material utilized includes radiopaque studies of living persons and surgical demonstrations of topographical relationships.

Scientific terms refer to position, portions, regions, and spaces of the body, including the head, neck, thorax, abdomen, pelvis, and upper and lower extremities. External anatomical positions include the following aspects: front, anterior (ventral); back, posterior (dorsal); and sides, lateral. Cross sections shown are midsagittal (along a line in the midline from front to back), sagittal (along any line parallel to midsagittal), horizontal or transverse (on a plane perpendicular to the sagittal plane), and frontal or coronal (on a plane from side to side). A view from above the head or toward the head is termed *cephalic* or *cephalad*. A view from below the coccyx or toward the coccyx is termed *caudal* or *caudad*. *Superior* is synonymous with *cephalic,* and *inferior* is synonymous with *caudal.*

Leon Schlossberg

Plate 1.
Anatomic Positions, Surface and Topographic Anatomy, and Regions and Planes of Sections

Cranium

Pleural cavities and lungs

Heart and pericardium

Thorax

Diaphragm

Abdomen

Upper extremity

Pelvis

Rectus abdominis

Umbilicus

Groin

Lower extremity

Anterior (ventral)

Deltoid

Inf. angle of scapula

Sacrospinalis

Iliac crest

Gluteus medius

Gluteus maximus

Posterior (dorsal)

Pectoralis major

Costal margin

Serratus ant.

Horizontal or transverse

Lateral

Suprasternal notch

Infrasternal notch

Ant.- sup. iliac spine

Midsagittal

Coronal or frontal

Epigastric

Lateral sternal

Parasternal

Midclavicular

Hypochondrium

Lumbar

Left lateral

Iliac

Umbilical

Inguinal lig.

Hypogastric

Transtubercular

Regions

Liver

Stomach

Spleen

Pancreas

Transverse colon

Descending colon

Gallbladder

Small intestine

Ascending colon

Cecum

Sigmoid colon

Ileum

Rectum

Appendix

The Johns Hopkins Atlas of Human Functional Anatomy

Fetal Circulation

John J. White, M.D.

1

in the decidua basalis, the maternal contribution to the placenta. On the fetal side of the placenta, a similar network of end vessels is elaborated in the chorionic villi.

The two circulations, maternal uterine and fetal, remain separate. The spaces between them are called *intervillous spaces* (see Plate 2, detail). Nutrients provided by the maternal circulation diffuse across the uterine capillary membrane, to be picked up, across the membranes of the umbilical capillary network, by the fetal circulation. Similarly, oxygen is taken up by the fetus and carbon dioxide is released.

From the placenta, the oxygen-rich, nutritious blood is delivered to the fetus by the umbilical vein in the umbilical cord. Upon entry to the fetus at the umbilicus, the umbilical vein travels to the liver, where it divides into two branches. A lesser portion of the blood supplies the liver, via the sinus intermedius. Most of the oxygenated and nutrient-rich blood passes through the liver, via the ductus venosus, to the inferior vena cava and the right heart. In the right atrium it mixes somewhat with cephalic venous blood of the fetus and is then shunted past the nonfunctional fetal lungs by two pathways basically. In the heart, most of the oxygenated blood flows through an opening between the two atria, the foramen ovale, into the left heart for distribution to the entire body (red arrows). Most of the unoxygenated fetal venous blood flows from the right atrium into the right ventricle and pulmonary artery (blue arrows). At this point another shunt, the ductus arteriosus, allows this blood to flow into the descending aorta, bypassing the brain and heart. Deoxygenated and nutrient-depleted blood from the fetus flows via major branch vessels of the aorta, the paired internal iliac or hypogastric arteries, back to the umbilicus, where these arteries pass, in the cord as the umbilical arteries, back to the placenta.

With and immediately after birth, physiologic processes active in the mother and baby bring about changes from the fetal-placental circulation to the normal extrauterine circulatory state. Respiratory activity of the neonate clears fluid from the lungs, aerates and inflates the alveoli, and stimulates active blood flow in the pulmonary vessels. As the pulmonary vascular resistance lowers, the decreased pressure at the ductus arteriosus decreases its size; functionally, it generally closes shortly after birth. As the pressure in the left atrium builds up with blood return from the lungs, the foramen ovale also closes functionally. This is abetted by diminished pressure in the right atrium as the ductus venosus also ceases to shunt blood through the liver. The hypogastric arteries obliterate back to the internal iliacs, which then only supply the pelvis.

The basic requirements for human life are nutrition and respiration. These requirements are even more special in the fetus, which, starting from the union of two germ cells and emerging forty weeks later as a neonate, must undergo formation, development, and growth. The requirements in question are provided in utero via the fetal circulatory system.

During its entire intrauterine existence, the fetus is, in effect, a parasite dependent completely upon its mother for its nutrition and respiration. Shortly after embryogenesis begins, the essence of the fetal circulatory system is formed by the placental-umbilical circulation. The placenta, an organ that is made up of both fetal and maternal uterine contributory parts, adheres firmly to the inner wall of the uterus. On the maternal side, the uterine circulation hypertrophies significantly, and specialized end vessels elaborate

Plate 2.
Fetal Circulation

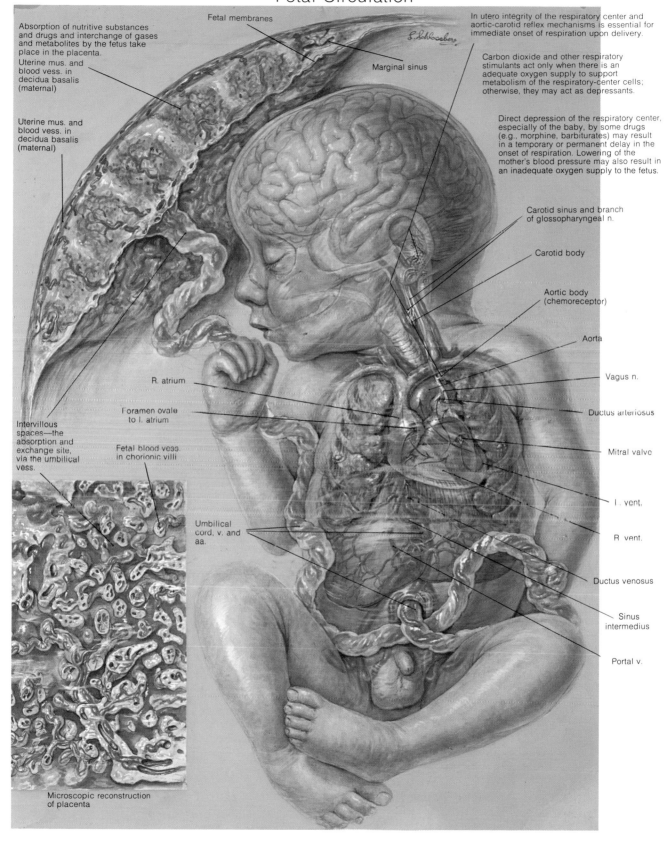

Absorption of nutritive substances and drugs and interchange of gases and metabolites by the fetus take place in the placenta.

Uterine mus. and blood vess. in decidua basalis (maternal)

Uterine mus. and blood vess. in decidua basalis (maternal)

Fetal membranes

Marginal sinus

In utero integrity of the respiratory center and aortic-carotid reflex mechanisms is essential for immediate onset of respiration upon delivery.

Carbon dioxide and other respiratory stimulants act only when there is an adequate oxygen supply to support metabolism of the respiratory-center cells; otherwise, they may act as depressants.

Direct depression of the respiratory center, especially of the baby, by some drugs (e.g., morphine, barbiturates) may result in a temporary or permanent delay in the onset of respiration. Lowering of the mother's blood pressure may also result in an inadequate oxygen supply to the fetus.

Carotid sinus and branch of glossopharyngeal n.

Carotid body

Aortic body (chemoreceptor)

Aorta

Vagus n.

Ductus arteriosus

Mitral valve

L. vent.

R. vent.

Ductus venosus

Sinus intermedius

Portal v.

R. atrium

Foramen ovale to l. atrium

Intervillous spaces—the absorption and exchange site, via the umbilical vess.

Fetal blood vess. in chorionic villi

Umbilical cord, v. and aa.

Microscopic reconstruction of placenta

Skeletal Anatomy

James L. Hughes, M.D.

2

The skeletal system is formed from bone, a complex, specialized connective tissue. Bone has many unique properties that enable it to carry out a diversity of functions. It performs a mechanical function in providing for the skeletal support of the body, in protecting the vital organs of the cranial and thoracic cavities, and in providing the platform for the attachment of muscles. The structure of bone is beautifully adapted to its various roles by utilizing the least material in association with the least weight that will enable it to function properly. Bone is engineered like reinforced concrete, with the collagen fibers resembling steel rods and the calcium the concrete itself.

Bone is active metabolically and provides for the immediate calcium needs of the body. The blood calcium concentration is maintained at a steady level by the reciprocal activity of parathyroid hormone and thyrocalcitonin on the bone cells. These cells regulate bone matrix and bone mineral (hydroxyapatite crystals) formation and resorption. Bone mineral can be added or removed from the matrix, depending on the body's need for calcium. In the normal adult, the formed elements of the blood—red cells, white cells, and platelets—originate in the bone marrow cavity. The principal source of these hematopoietic cells is the long bones (red marrow), while the marrow cavities (yellow marrow) of many other bones exist as reserve sites in the time of need.

Macroscopically, bone is either cancellous (spongy) or compact. Cancellous bone is primarily formed in the flat bones of the body—that is, in the cranium, pelvis, vertebrae, and scapula—and is rapidly responsive to metabolic exchanges. The cancellous bone occupies significant space in the skeleton, but it accounts for only one-fifth of the mass of bone. Both cancellous and compact bone consist of the same materials but differ in their architecture. Cancellous bone is arranged in trabeculae (thin plates), while compact bone is arranged in a lamellar pattern formed by concentric layers of bone fibers. This arrangement of fibers in lamellar bone provides maximum strength; thus, lamellar bone is found primarily in the long bones, which are constantly under stress.

Lamellar bone consists of numerous Haversian systems. A Haversian system, or osteon, consists of a central blood vessel, bone cells, and lamellar bone.

Microscopically, the greatest part of the mass of bone is made up of bone matrix. Embedded within this matrix are lacunae (cavities), which are completely filled with bone cells called *osteocytes*. Originating from the lacunae are small canals called *canaliculi*, which penetrate the hard interstitial substance in all directions. These canals branch and communicate with each other in such a manner as to connect all the lacunae together. The presence of this network of canals, plus the fact that no bone cell is more than 0.1 mm from a capillary, guarantees that every cell in bone is nourished and viable.

Remodeling and rebuilding of bone is accomplished by cells found on the surface of bone, the osteoclasts and osteoblasts. All three types of bone cells arise from a common stem cell, and transformation from one to the other is frequent. The activities of these cells enable a fractured bone to heal and remodel in accordance with the stresses applied to it.

In a typical long bone, such as the femur, the diaphysis (shaft) consists of compact bone surrounding a large cavity (medullary cavity) housing the bone marrow. The ends of the long bones are called *epiphyses* and consist of cancellous bone surrounded by a thin layer of cortical bone. In a growing child, the diaphysis is separated from the epiphysis by the epiphyseal cartilage plate. This area of trabecular bone and cartilage plate is sometimes called the *metaphysis* and permits growth in length of the long bones. In the flat bones of the skull, the compact bone is present on the inner and outer surfaces, between which is a layer of spongy bone called the *diploë.*

All bones are covered with a specialized form of connective tissue called *periosteum,* with a somewhat similar tissue called the *endosteum* lining the marrow spaces. These layers are quite thick in the growing child, as they furnish the cells providing for bone growth and remodeling. As the aging process occurs, the layers become thinner but are never completely abolished.

Bones are joined to one another by joints, which allow varying degrees of motion between adjoining bones. These are quite variable in nature. Some articulations, such as between two bones of the skull, allow for no motion; these are called *synarthroses.* There are three types of these, named for the tissue connecting the two bones: bone (synostosis), cartilage (synchondrosis), and connective tissue (syndesmosis). Joints that allow free movement of the bones are called *diarthroses.* An example of a diarthrodial joint is the knee. This type of joint surrounds the articular ends of long bones, which are covered with hyaline cartilage. These joints have a capsule that consists of a dense, fibrous outer layer (fibrous layer) and a cellular, inner layer (synovial layer). This synovial layer secretes the liquid (synovia) that lubricates the joint surfaces. The cartilage lining the surfaces of the bone within the joint has no blood supply with which to nourish itself; this function is performed by the synovial fluid.

The skeleton is usually considered to have two main divisions: the axial skeleton, which includes the skull, vertebral column, sternum, and ribs; and the appendicular skeleton, which includes the limbs, shoulders, and pelvic girdle.

The skull is composed of a series of flat, irregular bones that, except for the mandible, are immovably joined together. It can be divided into two units: the cranium, which protects the brain and which consists of eight bones; and the skeleton of the face, which includes fourteen bones.

The cranium consists of the frontal, occipital, sphenoid, ethmoid, two parietal, and two temporal bones. On viewing the skull from the side, we see that the frontal bone forms the anterior wall and the occipital bone the posterior wall. The parietal bones form the superior lateral walls, and the temporal bones form the lower lateral walls. The sphenoid bone forms the floor of the cranial vault, joining anteriorly with the frontal bone and posteriorly with the occipital bone. The foramen magnum, a large opening through which the spinal cord passes, is present in the occipital bone. Two bony protuberances, called *condyles,* are present next to the foramen magnum. These structures articulate with the cervical spine, allowing for flexion and extension motions of the head. Ten pairs of major foramina and fissures are present in the skull, allowing for passage of nerves and blood vessels.

The vertebral column is a flexible unit that gives support to the cranium, provides an attachment for the ribs, protects the spinal column, and provides for muscle attachments. Viewed laterally, it has four curves, two convex and two concave. The concave curves are found in the thoracic and sacrococcygeal areas, while the convex curves are in the cervical and lumbar regions. The alternating curves provide for increased weight-bearing strength of the column.

The spine is composed of thirty-three bones, the vertebrae, which are classified as follows: seven cervical, twelve thoracic, five lumbar, five sacral, and four coccygeal. In the adult, the sacral and coccygeal vertebrae are fused into two bones, the sacrum and the coccyx. Although the vertebrae differ in size, they are basically similar in structure. Each has a body that supports weight, a neural axis that protects the spinal cord, a spinous process and a right and left transverse process, all of which provide for muscle attachments, and four articular processes, which control movement. The first two cervical vertebrae, the atlas and the axis, are specialized, providing for attachment and movement of the cranium. The intervertebral disc lies between adjacent vertebrae.

The thorax is a cage that is composed of twelve ribs on each side, which are attached to the vertebrae in back. The upper seven pairs of ribs are called the "true" ribs, for they attach directly to the sternum, whereas the lower five pairs are the "false" ribs, for their attachments anteriorly are either free (ribs 11 and 12) or to the cartilages of the preceding ribs (ribs 8, 9, and 10). The sternum is composed of the manubrium, body, and xiphoid process.

The bones by which the upper extremities are attached to the skeleton are called the *shoulder girdle,* and consist of the scapula posteriorly and the clavicle anteriorly. In the shoulder, only the clavicle is firmly attached to the skeleton by its articulation with the sternum, whereas the scapula is free-floating, surrounded only by muscles. This anatomical arrangement allows for a wide and varied arc of motion. The scapula is a triangular, flat bone with three borders, two surfaces, and three angles. The scapular spine is a prominent, raised area posteriorly that terminates laterally in the acromion. The acromion forms the summit of the shoulder and provides for the attachment of the clavicle at the acromioclavicular

Plate 3.
The Skull

1. Supraorbital for.
2. Optic for.
3. Sup. orbital fissure
4. Rotundum for.
5. Inf. orbital fissure
6. Ant. lacrimal ridge
7. Fossa for lacrimal sac
8. Infraorbital foramen and groove
9. Nasal cavity and inf. concha
10. Mandible
11. Condyle
12. Coronoid
13. Mandibular for. and lingula
14. Mental for.
15. Mylohyoid groove
16. Frontal sinus
17. Openings of maxillary sinus
18. Maxillary sinus
19. Pterygoid hamulus
20. Openings of post. ethmoid cells
21. Sphenopalatine for.
22. Sphenoid sinus and opening into nose
23. Sup. concha
24. Nasal bone
25. Middle concha and openings of nasofrontal duct and ant. ethmoid cells

26. Bulla ethmoidalis (openings of middle ethmoid cells
27. Inf. concha and opening of nasolacrimal duct
28. Incisive for.
29. For. cecum
30. Crista galli and olfactory n. for.
31. Greater and lesser palatine for.
32. Zygomatic arch
33. Nasal septum
34. Ant. clinoid
35. Pituitary fossa
36. For. ovale
37. Post. clinoid
38. For. spinosum and groove for middle meningeal a.
39. For. lacerum
40. Orifice for Eustachian tube
41. For. carotid
42. Ext. auditory meatus
43. Styloid process
44. Jugular fossa
45. Occipital condyle and fossa
46. Mastoid process and stylomastoid for.
47. Petrous portion temporal bone and groove for sup. petrosal sinus

48. Int. auditory meatus
49. Hypoglossal canal
50. Jugular foramen
51. Foramen magnum
52. Mastoid foramen
53. Groove for occipital sinus
54. Groove for transverse sinus
55. Groove for sup. sagittal sinus
56. Orbit
57. Ant. and middle ethmoid cells
58. Middle concha
59. Inf. concha
60. Nasal floor
61. Ant. ethmoid cells
62. Post ethmoid cells
63. Lamina papyracea

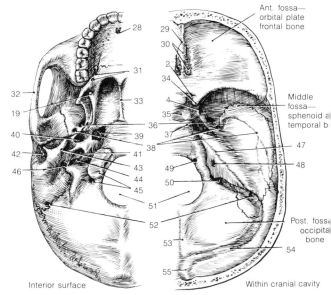

BASE OF SKULL

Interior surface · Within cranial cavity

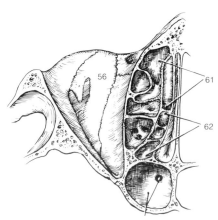

joint. On the lateral aspect of the scapula is a rounded, concave area, called the *glenoid cavity,* which articulates proximally with the largest bone of the upper extremity, the humerus.

In the humeral head is a constricted area called the *anatomical neck,* whereas a constriction just below the greater and lesser tubercles, which is frequently the site of fracture, is termed the *surgical neck.* Articulation with the forearm is accomplished laterally through the capitulum with the radial head and medially through the trochlea with the ulna. These articulations allow two types of movements in the elbow, flexion-extension and pronation-supination. The radius, which lies laterally in the forearm, widens distally to form the major articulation with the carpal bones. The wrist is composed of eight small carpal bones, and the hand is made up of five metacarpal bones and fourteen phalanges.

The pelvic girdle is formed by the articulation of the two innominate bones posteriorly to the sacrum and anteriorly to each other through an articulation called the *symphysis pubis.* The innominate bones themselves are actually a fusion of three bones, the ischium, pubis, and ilium. Laterally, these three bones meet and form a saucerlike confluence called the *acetabulum,* which articulates with the femoral head forming the hip joint.

The femur, the longest and strongest bone in the body, is proximally divided into the femoral head and neck and the greater and lesser trochanters. The trochanters provide for the attachment of some of the muscles utilized in hip movement and are frequently the sites of fractures. Distally, the femur expands into a large medial and lateral condyle for articulation with the proximal tibia. An anterior concavity between the condyles allows for patella movement.

The tibia and fibula are the bones of the lower leg. The tibia is a triangular-shaped bone whose sharp anterior edge is known as the *shin.* Distally, the tibia and fibula form, respectively, the medial and lateral malleoli, which, with the talus, form the ankle joint.

The bony structure of the foot is similar to that of the hand. The seven tarsal bones articulate with five metatarsals. The phalanges number fourteen. The bones of the foot are bound together by ligaments, muscles, and tendons into two arches, one longitudinal and one transverse. These arches allow for the flexibility necessary in walking.

Plate 4.
Skeleton—Anterior and Posterior Views

64. Ext. occipital protuberance
65. Acromion
66. Coracoid process
67. Glenoid cavity
68. Spine
69. Inf. angle
70. Vert. and axillary borders
71. Costal cart.
72. Greater tubercle
73. Lesser tubercle
74. Head
75. Lat. epicondyle
76. Med. epicondyle
77. Trochlea
78. Capitulum
79. Coronoid fossa
80. Radial fossa
81. Olecranon
82. Coronoid process

Frontal
Orbital plate
Nasal
Lacrimal plate
Zygomatic
Clavicle
1st rib
Manubrium
Scapula
Sternum
Xiphoid
Humerus
Vertebra
Intervertebral disc
12th rib
Sacral foramina
Radius
Ulna
Navicular
Capitate
Greater multangular
Lesser multangular
Metacarpal
Phalanges
Pisiform
Triangular
Hamate
Lunate
Femur
Patella
Tibia
Fibula

Pelvis
Sacrum
Coccyx

Anatomical Position
Arm in supination to demonstrate
details of anatomy

Physiological Position
Note that only a portion of the
head of the humerus is in
relation to the glenoid fossa
of the scapula.

Clavicle
Acromion
Scapula
Olecranon in
olecranon fossa
Pelvis
Sacrum
Coccyx
Talus
Metatarsal
Calcaneus
Cuboid

83. Head
84. Neck
85. Radial tuberosity
86. Styloid processes
87. Crest of ilium
88. Ant., sup., and inf. spines
89. Spine of ischium
90. Tuberosity of ischium
91. Symphysis pubis
92. Obturator foramen
93. Inf. ramus of pubis
94. Sup. ramus of pubis
    and pubic tubercle
95. Post., sup., and inf. spines
96. Greater sciatic notch
97. Sacral and coccygeal cornua
98. Sacral hiatus leading to
    caudal canal
99. Head of femur in acetabulum
100. Greater trochanter
101. Lesser trochanter
102. Neck
103. Intertrochanteric line
104. Intertrochanteric crest
105. Lat. epicondyle
106. Med. epicondyle
107. Adductor tubercle
108. Tuberosity
109. Med. malleolus
110. Lat. malleolus
111. Trans. process, pedicle, foramen,
     and groove for spinal n.

Plate 5.
Skeleton—Lateral View

Temporal

Parietal

Sphenoid

64

Hyoid bone

1-7 cervical vert.

111

113

114

112

Body of 6th cervical vert.

117

111

115

116

114

Vertebra

Vertebral column

Intervertebral disc

118

113

Rib cage

118   115

113

114

119

120

Body of 6th thoracic vert.

1-12 thoracic vert.

121

116

122

1-5 lumbar vert.

Femur

Sacrum

Coccyx

118

113

114

115

Body of 4th lumbar vert.

Patella

108

Talus

Calcaneus

Navicular

1st cuneiform

2nd cuneiform

3rd cuneiform

Cuboid

Metatarsal

Phalanges

Tibia

Fibula

110

112. Vertebral foramen
113. Lamina
114. Spinous process
115. Sup. articular facet
116. Inf. articular facet
117. Odontoid process
118. Transverse process
119. Demi-facet for head of rib
120. Facet for articular part of
     tubercle of rib
121. Intervertebral foramen for
     spinal n.
122. Pedicle

Skeletal Muscles, Joints, and Fascial Structures

3

Vernon Tolo, M.D.

The essential feature of muscle, which leads to movement in all parts of the body, is its ability to contract. Unlike smooth muscle or cardiac muscle, skeletal, or striated, muscle contracts only under nerve control, i.e., voluntarily or reflexly. This muscle type accounts for about 40 percent of human body weight. Although Leonardo da Vinci in his classic anatomic drawings used letters to designate specific muscles, and Galen and Vesalius used numbers for this purpose, muscles are currently referred to by names. These names may describe the function, direction, or attachment of the muscles, or may simply describe the shape, size, or structure of the specific muscle.

Muscles are composed of multiple bundles of fibers. Hypertrophy of existing muscle fibers occurs with muscle training, but there is no way to increase the number of muscle fibers. Muscle must be stressed to work effectively, and inactivity or bedrest leads to a loss of muscle size and strength.

The muscle attachments are usually designated the origin and the insertion. The origin is located proximally and near the midline, while the insertion is the distal, peripheral attachment. These attachments bridge one or more joints, and the result of muscle contraction is joint movement. The principal actions of muscles are fourfold. A prime mover muscle effects the actual movement that occurs. An antagonist acts by relaxing to enable the prime mover to work, and the antagonist is capable, by contraction, of preventing the movement. A fixation muscle provides a stable base by steadying a part of the body from which other muscles perform, and a synergistic muscle controls the position of intermediate joints so that the prime movers passing over several joints may exert power in moving the distal joint.

Each group of several fibers receives a nerve supply that allows voluntary contraction of the muscle. Initiated in the cerebral cortex, the stimulus for voluntary muscle action passes down the spinal cord and the nerve root to the motor end-plate, the junction of the nerve with the muscle fibers. Release of acetylcholine at the motor end-plate allows transmission of the stimulus from the nerve to the muscle, resulting in the contraction of the muscle fibers. When a muscle contracts, all fibers innervated by the stimulated motor end-plate contract either fully or not at all, with increasing numbers of fibers recruited as the work load becomes heavier. During muscle action, the basic microscopic muscle unit, the sarcomere, shortens. The energy for the contraction of the muscle is obtained primarily from free fatty acids, glucose, or glycogen. Muscles requiring rapid movement largely contain white, or fast, fibers high in glycogen content, and muscles doing sustained, heavier work are of the red, or slow, fiber type. These fiber groups are found in varying amounts in different muscles depending on the primary muscle function.

Prolongations of the muscles at the insertion are called *tendons,* collagenous tissue bands that obviate the need for long muscle fibers, decrease the bulk of tissue around the joints, and provide protection against muscle injury during sudden movement of the joint. Many tendons are enclosed in a synovial sheath, a fascial structure that provides smoother motion and nutrition for the tendons.

Fascial structures are present throughout the body and are derived from the mesoderm, the same embryonic tissue from which muscles arise. Superficial fascia, lying just beneath the skin, is impregnated with fat of differing degrees. Because of its areolar quality, this layer is particularly subject to edema following limb injury. The deep fascia is a thick fibrous membrane that encloses muscles, blends with the ligaments, and attaches to bony surfaces. By forming intermuscular septa, the deep fascia separates groups of muscles or individual muscles. By forming retinaculae at the wrist and ankle, it keeps the tendons in position and acts as a pulley for tendon action. The synovial sheaths are localized thickenings of the deep fascia to facilitate tendon movement. Bursae are sacs of synovial tissue that develop between a moving tendon and a bony prominence or ligament over which the tendon passes. They are usually located near joints. Bursitis, the inflammation of these structures, is a common ailment in the shoulder, elbow, and knee after excessive or unusual activity of these joints.

Joints are the articulations between adjacent bones. The majority of the joints of the extremities are synovial joints, which are specialized to allow free movement. The synovium lines the joint cavity and secretes synovial fluid to nourish smooth, avascular articular cartilage covering the ends of the articulating bones. The articulating bones remain opposed by muscle tension and the strength of ligaments bridging the joints. Ligaments are fibrous tissue bands that cross a joint and change lengths with joint movement. They do not voluntarily contract or relax. Ligaments attach bone to bone, whereas tendons attach muscle to bones. Two common joint types are the hinge joint (elbow, knee, and finger) and the ball-and-socket joint (hip and shoulder).

NECK AND TRUNK MUSCLES

The axial muscles of the neck and trunk are innervated by spinal nerves and are segmentally arranged. The largest muscles involved with neck movements are the sternomastoid and the trapezius. Additional anterior neck muscles are the longus colli, scalenus anterior, scalenus medius, scalenus posterior, rectus capitis, and longus capitis. The platysma muscle, with a role in facial expression, lies anteriorly in the region of the superficial fascia. Swallowing, speech, and chewing involve the muscles in the laryngeal and esophageal regions called *strap* muscles, which include the omohyoid, sternohyoid, sternothyroid, thyrohyoid, digastric, stylohyoid, mylohyoid, and geniohyoid muscles.

The most important muscle in the thorax is the diaphragm, the principal muscle for respiration. Assisting the diaphragm in respiration are the external and internal intercostal muscles. Other thoracic muscles are the transversus thoracis, subcostals, levatores costarum, and serrati posteriores. The abdominal wall muscles, discussed in Chapter Four, occur in several layers with the principal ones being the external oblique, internal oblique, transversus abdominus, and rectus abdominus muscle. The muscles of the back are arranged in three layers: the erector spinae system, the transversospinalis system, and the deep layer. The erector spinae group, consisting of the spinalis thoracis, longissimus, splenius capitis, and erector spinae muscles, run longitudinally and span several vertebrae. The transversospinalis system runs obliquely and consists of the multifidus and semispinalis muscle groups. These usually span fewer vertebrae. The deep layer includes the interspinalis, intertransverse, and suboccipital muscles, which span only adjacent vertebrae. The disabling effect of low back pain visibly demonstrates the interplay necessary between these multiple muscles if smooth functioning of the back is to occur. Asymmetrical function of the back muscles, particularly in neuromuscular diseases, may lead to scoliosis, a lateral curvature of the spine.

The most distal trunk muscles are those of the pelvic diaphragm and perineum. Necessary because of the erect posture in humans, the pelvic diaphragm holds up the pelvic floor and consists of the coccygeus and levator ani, formed by the iliococcygeus and pubococcygeus muscles. In the perineum, the anal triangle, located posteriorly, contains the sphincter ani externus; the urogenital triangle, situated anteriorly, contains the superficial transversus perinei, bulbospongiosus, ischiocavernosus, sphincter urethrae, and the deep transverse perineal muscles. The perineal body connects the anal and urogenital triangles.

Another upper trunk muscle group serves to connect the upper limb to the trunk. These muscles are responsible for scapular and clavicular motion as a part of upper extremity movement. The dorsal muscles are the trapezius, levator scapuli, rhomboids, and the latissimus dorsi, the widest muscle of the back. The ventral or anterior muscles are the pectoralis major, pectoralis minor, subclavius, and serratus anterior. Although the principal action of these muscles is involved with shoulder girdle motion, stabilization of the upper extremities will allow the reverse action to occur, and the pectoralis major and minor, latissimus dorsi, trapezius, and sternomastoid muscles can all work as accessory respiratory muscles.

UPPER EXTREMITY MUSCLES AND JOINTS

The shoulder, a ball-and-socket joint with the widest range of motion of any joint in the body, has freedom of motion at the expense of stability and is the most easily dislocated of the major joints. The shoulder girdle moves at the articulation between the humerus and glenoid cavity of the scapula, but the scapula also moves on the chest wall and the clavicle rotates at its joints. In abduction of the shoulder, for exam-

Plate 6.
Muscles, Ligaments and Fasciae, Tendons, and Bursae—Anterior View

Orbicularis oculi
Zygomaticus
Risorius
Ant., middle, and post. scaleni
Sternomastoid
Platysma
Subclavius
Pectoralis major
Deltoid
Pectoralis minor
Subscapularis
Triceps brachii
Biceps
Brachioradialis
Pronator teres
Lacertus fibrosus
Flexor carpi radialis
Flexor carpi ulnaris
Palmaris longus

Frontal
Orbicularis oris
Temporal
Buccinator
Longus coli
Trapezius
Coracoacromial
Subacromial
Subdeltoid
Subcoracoid
Articular capsule
Coracobrachialis
Teres major
Biceps (long head)
Latissimus dorsi
Biceps (short head)
Serratus ant.
Ext. and int. intercostal
Brachialis
Int. oblique

Post. rectus sheath
Rectus abdominis
Inguinal
Trochanteric
Iliopectineal
Iliac
Iliopsoas
Obturator externus
Adductor minimus
Pyramidalis
Adductor magnus
Adductor canal (Hunter's)
Pectineus
Adductor longus
Fibular collateral
Lat. meniscus
Suprapatellar
Adductor magnus
Patellar
Med. meniscus
Peroneus
Tibial collateral
Ext. hallucis longus

Tensor fasciae latae
Inguinal
Sartorius
Vastus lateralis
Rectus femoris
Gracilis
Vastus medialis
Pre- and infrapatellar
Peroneus longus
Gastrocnemius
Ant. tibial
Peroneus brevis
Ext. digitorum longus
Trans. crural

Patella
Soleus
Cruciate crural

Abductor pollicis brevis
Radial a.
Ulnar a.
Trans. carpal
Ulnar bursa
Radial bursa (flexor pollicis longus)
Hypothenar cleft
Middle palmar cleft
Flexor pollicis brevis
Lumbrical clefts
Thenar cleft
Sheath of flexor digitorum, sublimis and profundus

Dorsal carpal
Ext. carpi radialis longus
Abductor pollicis longus
Ext. pollicis brevis
Abductor pollicis brevis
Ext. pollicis longus
Interosseous
Lumbrical
Flexor digitorum sublimis
Flexor digitorum profundus
Sheath
Retinaculum
Vincula longa
Ext. digitorum communis
First lumbrical
First dorsal Interosseous

Plate 7.
Muscles, Ligaments and Fasciae, Tendons, and Bursae—Posterior View

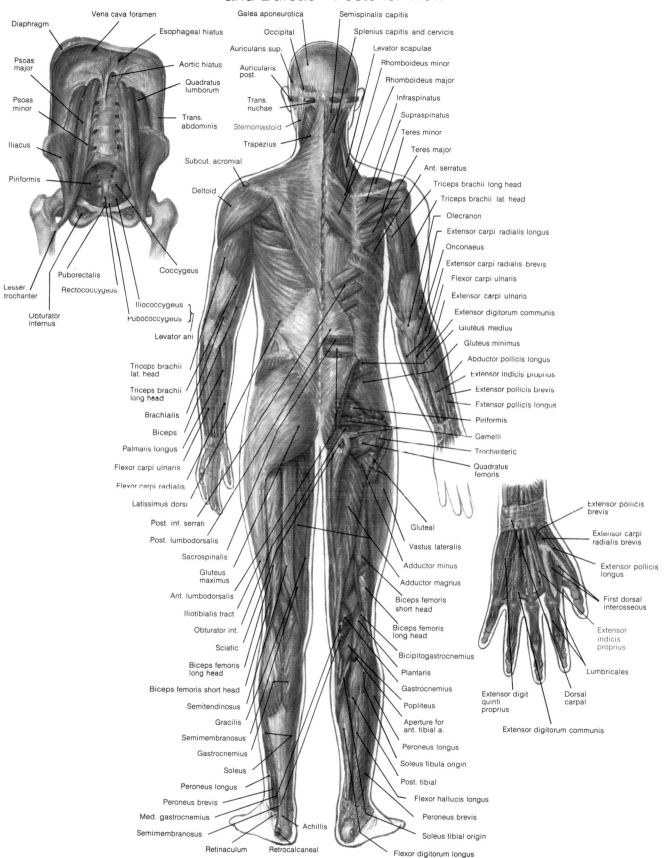

Diaphragm
Vena cava foramen
Galea aponeurotica
Semispinalis capitis
Esophageal hiatus
Occipital
Splenius capitis and cervicis
Psoas major
Auricularis sup.
Levator scapulae
Aortic hiatus
Auricularis post.
Rhomboideus minor
Quadratus lumborum
Rhomboideus major
Psoas minor
Trans. nuchae
Infraspinatus
Trans. abdominis
Sternomastoid
Supraspinatus
Iliacus
Trapezius
Teres minor
Teres major
Subcut. acromial
Ant. serratus
Piriformis
Triceps brachii long head
Deltoid
Triceps brachii lat. head
Olecranon
Extensor carpi radialis longus
Onconaeus
Extensor carpi radialis brevis
Flexor carpi ulnaris
Puborectalis
Extensor carpi ulnaris
Coccygeus
Extensor digitorum communis
Lesser trochanter
Rectococcygeus
Gluteus medius
Obturator internus
Iliococcygeus
Gluteus minimus
Pubococcygeus
Abductor pollicis longus
Levator ani
Extensor Indicis proprius
Extensor pollicis brevis
Triceps brachii lat. head
Extensor pollicis longus
Triceps brachii long head
Piriformis
Brachialis
Gemelli
Biceps
Trochanteric
Palmaris longus
Quadratus femoris
Flexor carpi ulnaris
Flexor carpi radialis
Latissimus dorsi
Extensor pollicis brevis
Post. int. serrati
Gluteal
Post. lumbodorsalis
Extensor carpi radialis brevis
Vastus lateralis
Sacrospinalis
Extensor pollicis longus
Gluteus maximus
Adductor minus
Ant. lumbodorsalis
Adductor magnus
First dorsal interosseous
Iliotibialis tract
Biceps femoris short head
Obturator int.
Extensor indicis proprius
Sciatic
Biceps femoris long head
Biceps femoris long head
Bicipitogastrocnemius
Lumbricales
Biceps femoris short head
Plantaris
Extensor digit quinti proprius
Semitendinosus
Gastrocnemius
Dorsal carpal
Gracilis
Popliteus
Extensor digitorum communis
Semimembranosus
Aperture for ant. tibial a.
Gastrocnemius
Peroneus longus
Soleus
Soleus fibula origin
Peroneus longus
Post. tibial
Peroneus brevis
Flexor hallucis longus
Med. gastrocnemius
Peroneus brevis
Semimembranosus
Achillis
Soleus tibial origin
Retinaculum
Retrocalcaneal
Flexor digitorum longus

ple, approximately two-thirds of this abduction results from movement between the glenoid and the humeral head, while one-third comes from rotation of the scapula on the chest wall. The glenoid is approximately one-third the surface of the humeral head. What strength and stability of the joint is present results from the attachments of muscles close to the articular surface. The least joint support occurs inferiorly, the direction in which dislocation most commonly occurs. Bursitis in the shoulder area is common. The subscapular bursa communicates with the joint, whereas the subacromial bursa, located below the deltoid, does not.

Numerous muscles interact in shoulder motion, as the shoulder joint is free to move in almost any plane. The deltoid and rotator cuff are the principal abductors of the shoulder. The rotator cuff, consisting of subscapularis, supraspinatus, infraspinatus, and teres minor, keep the articular surfaces together and initiate abduction, while the deltoid provides the major strength for continued abduction at the shoulder. Adduction and medial (internal) rotation of the shoulder are mediated by the pectoralis major, latissimus dorsi, and teres major. The infraspinatus and teres minor effect lateral rotation, while extension is performed by the latissimus dorsi and the posterior deltoid muscle. Flexion of the shoulder is mediated by the pectoralis major and the anterior deltoid fibers. The biceps and the triceps of the upper arm have separate origins, which cross over the shoulder joint but act weakly on shoulder motion per se.

The muscles of the upper arm are divided into anterior and posterior groups. The anterior group includes the coracobrachialis, brachialis, a pure flexor of the elbow, and biceps brachii, which functions primarily to supinate the forearm and secondarily to flex the elbow. The triceps brachii, for elbow extension, is posterior. The elbow is principally a hinge joint. The ulna articulates with the trochlea, while the radius articulates with the capitulum portion of the humerus. The collateral ligaments and muscles around the elbow augment the inherent stability of this joint provided by the bony contours of the humerus, ulna, and radius. The principal bursa in this area is that overlying the olecranon process of the ulna.

The muscles of the forearm form two groups. The anteromedial, flexor-pronator group is divided into three layers. The superficial layer has its origin on the medial humeral epicondyle and is formed by the pronator teres, flexor carpi radialis, palmaris longus, and flexor carpi ulnaris muscles. The second layer is formed by the flexor digitorum profundus, flexor pollicis longus, and, in the distal forearm, the pronator quadratus muscles. The posterolateral group forms two layers. The most superficial are the extensor carpi radialis longus, brachioradialis, anconeus, ex-

tensor carpi radialis brevis, extensor digitorum, extensor digiti minimi, and extensor carpi ulnaris. The last four muscles begin at the lateral humeral epicondyle; inflammation over this area constitutes "tennis elbow." The deep posterolateral layer is formed by the supinator, the abductor pollicis longus, the extensor pollicis brevis, extensor pollicis longus, and extensor indicis muscles. Movement at the wrist joint is principally in the plane of flexion and extension, but there is a complex interplay between the metacarpals, the eight carpal bones, and the distal radial and ulnar articulations.

The principal function of the upper extremity is to position the hand properly to do work or to guard or cover any part of the body. A major feature of human hand function is the ability to oppose the thumb to the digits. The interphalangeal joints of the hands are hinge joints, while the metacarpophalangeal joints allow some adduction and abduction as well as the hinge function. The first metacarpal joint is a saddle joint.

Movement of the hand is produced by a combination of the extrinsic muscles, originating in the forearm but inserting into the hand and wrist, and the shorter intrinsic muscles that arise within the hand itself. The thenar eminence consists of the abductor pollicis brevis, the opponens pollicis, and the flexor pollicis brevis muscles, all innervated by the median nerve. The adductor pollicis attaches deep to these muscles. The interosseous muscles include the palmar and dorsal groups. The four palmar interossei act as adductors from the hand at midline. The four dorsal interossei act as adductors from the midline with two muscular heads originating from adjacent metacarpal bones. The interossei muscles also flex the matacarpophalangeal joints and extend the interphalangeal joints. The four lumbrical muscles, associated closely with the flexor digitorum profundus tendons, are coordinated with the interossei for fine finger movements. The ulnar nerve innervates all the intrinsic muscles of the hand except the lateral two lumbricals and the thenar eminence muscles.

On the dorsum of the hand the skin is mobile, and swelling occurs in the superficial fascia here more readily than in the palmar aspect, where the skin is firmly bound to the underlying fascial structures. The arrangement of the deep fascia in the hand forms potential spaces, especially the mid-palmar space deep to the flexor tendons, where infection may occur. Other sites of potential infection are the tendon sheath of the flexor pollicis longus, the individual flexor sheaths of the second, third, and fourth fingers, and the ulnar bursa, or common flexor tendon sheath, which communicates with all flexor tendons except the thumb. Closed-space infections in these areas can destroy the lining of the synovial sheath and limit normal tendon motion.

Plate 8.
Shoulder and Hip Joints

LOWER EXTREMITIES MUSCLES AND JOINTS

The muscles and joints of the lower extremities provide strength and stability for the body. They serve to transmit the weight of the body and to provide locomotion of the body with an alternating, reciprocal gait. Postural balance must be maintained, and, depending on one's position, few or many of these muscles act reflexly to maintain balance. The action of these muscles when the trunk moves on fixed limbs differs from the action that occurs when the limbs move with the trunk fixed. When one is standing still, the primary lower extremity muscles that are acting are those of the calf.

The hip is a ball-and-socket joint. Because it is required to bear the body weight, the hip has a deep socket, a strong capsule, and muscular attachments at a distance from the movement axis—all different from comparable structures in the ball-and-socket joint at the shoulder. The labrum adds further stability at the lip of the acetabulum. The capsule of the hip is cylindrical and has obliquely running fibers. The hip capsule has the least capacity in an internal rotation position. With synovitis or inflammation of the hip joint, internal rotation motion is lost. A leg held externally rotated and fixed, the position in which the capsule has the largest capacity, generally indicates that hip inflammation or injury is present. Two thirds of the femoral neck is intracapsular, and with infection of the proximal femur, a secondary joint infection may occur from seepage through the bone. Another unique aspect of the hip is the arterial supply to the femoral head; the medial and lateral femoral circumflex arteries run through the capsule from distal to proximal, in this way making them prone to injury from surgery or trauma. The principal bursae around the hip are the greater trochanteric bursa, beneath the gluteus maximus tendon, and the lesser trochanteric bursa, beneath the psoas tendon.

The muscular structures around the hip are designed for strength and power, not finesse. Flexion of the hip is provided by the iliopsoas, with the iliacus arising in the pelvis and the psoas arising from the anterior lumbar spine. The rectus femoris and the sartorius cross both the hip and the knee joints and also act as hip flexors. The gluteus maximus, the heaviest muscle in the body, provides hip extension. This muscle is best developed in human beings because of their erect posture, and it is this muscle that forms the buttock shape. Hip abduction is mediated by the gluteus medius and gluteus minimus muscles. Weakness of these hip abductors through injury or disease will cause a waddling gait. External rotators of the hip include the piriformis, obturator internus, superior and inferior gemelli, and quadratus femoris muscles.

There are three primary groups of thigh muscles.

The posterior group, the hamstrings, are innervated by the sciatic nerve. The medial hamstrings are the semitendinous and semimembraneous muscles. The lateral hamstring is the biceps femoris. Because of the relative inelasticity of the hamstrings, originating on the ischial portion of the pelvis and attaching to the tibia, these muscles are a frequent source of injury in sports. The medial group, the adductors, are innervated by the obturator nerve. These muscles include the gracilis, adductor longus, adductor brevis, adductor magnus, pectineus, and obturator externus. The anterior group, the sartorius and the quadriceps femoris, are innervated by the femoral nerve and act as knee extensors. The sartorius in the longest muscle in the body. The quadriceps femoris is divided into the rectus femoris, which originates above the hip, and the vastus medialis, vastus intermedius, and vastus lateralis muscles. All the muscles of the quadriceps femoris coalesce distally to form the patellar ligament.

The knee, the largest joint in the body, is basically a modified hinge joint. Articulations are present between the tibia and the femur and between the patella and the femur. The patella is a sesamoid bone that is fully incorporated into the patellar tendon; it acts as a fulcrum to improve the quadriceps power during knee extension. The knee capsule is formed by a fibrous tissue extension from the muscle, and, because of its proximal muscle attachment, this capsule allows knee flexibility as well as stability. Four principal ligaments are present in the knee: medial and lateral collateral, and anterior and posterior cruciate ligaments. The lateral collateral ligament is closely associated with the iliotibial band, which is tightened proximally by the tensor fascia femoris muscle. The cruciate ligaments prevent anterior and posterior displacement of the tibia on the femur. The two menisci, wedge shaped in cross section, allow more even distribution of weight over the articular cartilage surfaces at the knee joint and may aid in lubrication of the articular surfaces. The lateral meniscus is O-shaped and the medial meniscus is a C-shaped structure. The medial meniscus is frequently torn in conjunction with medial collateral ligament injuries in sports. Because the menisci are avascular, a tear of these structures generally necessitates surgical removal because the scar tissue that forms remains weak and liable to reinjury. Medial rotation of the knee is effected by the popliteus muscle and by the sartorious, gracilis, and semitendinous muscles, which form the pes anserinus tendon at its insertion on the proximal medial tibia.

The fascia lata in the thigh, overlying the thigh muscles, is thin medially but thick laterally, forming the iliotibial band. Its proximal attachment is the tensor fascia femoris muscle, while its insertion aids in lateral knee stability. The lateral intermuscular sep-

Plate 9.
Knee Joint

Femur

Tendon of quadriceps femoris

Tendon of intermedius m.

Retinaculum from vastus medialis

Fibular collateral lig.

Capsular lig. of joint

Patellar lig.

Pes anserinus (tendons of sartorius, gracilis and semitendinosus)

Tibial tuberosity

Fibula

Tibial collateral lig.

Patella reflected upward

Femoral condyles

Post. cruciate lig.

Articular capsule (cutaway) { Fibrous stratum, Synovial stratum }

Synovial cavity

Articular cart.

Lat. meniscus

Med. meniscus

Ant. cruciate lig.

Lat. meniscus

Transverse lig.

Fibula   Tibia

Femur

Tibia

FRONTAL SECTION THROUGH MID FEMUR AND TIBIA

Suprapatellar bursa and communication with synovial cavity

Quadriceps tendon

Articular capsule { Cut edge of fibrous stratum, Synovial stratum (sac) }

Patella

Prepatellar bursa

Popliteal tendon

Infrapatellar fat pad

Fibular collateral lig.

Patellar lig.

Lat. meniscus

Infrapatellar bursa

Fibula

Tibia

Subcutaneous bursa

Femoral

Femur

Branch from deep femoral

Sup. genicular

Sup. med. genicular

Sup. lat. genicular

Popliteal

Inf. med. genicular

Inf. lat. genicular

Tibia

Recurrent a. from ant. tibial

Post. tibial

Fibula

Peroneal

ARTERIES AS SEEN FROM BEHIND

tum extends to the linea aspera of the entire femur and is attached to the fascia lata, while the medial intermuscular septum is present principally only in the distal third of the femur. The primary bursae in the area of the knee are the prepatella bursa and the infrapatella bursa, although the pes anserinus tendon frequently has a bursa beneath it.

Below the knee, four compartments are formed in the leg by the deep fascial attachments. The anterior compartment is composed of the tibialis anterior, the extensor digitorum longus, and the extensor hallicis longus muscles. The lateral compartment contains the peroneus longus and the peroneus brevis muscles. These extensor muscles of the anterior and lateral compartments are innervated by the peroneal nerve. Posterior to the tibia and fibula, the deep posterior compartment consists of the tibialis posterior, flexor hallucis longus, and flexor digitorum communis muscles; the posterior compartment contains the soleus, gastrocnemius, and plantaris muscles. These two compartments are innervated by the posterior tibial nerve. The flexor hallucis longus is a principal muscle for push-off in running or walking. The gastrocnemius and soleus compose the triceps surae and join distally to attach to the calcaneus as the Achilles tendon, the strongest tendon in the body. The gastrocnemius muscle originates above the knee, whereas the soleus originates below the knee.

The ankle joint is a hinge joint and functions to transfer weight through the tibia to the talus. The lateral collateral ligaments of the ankle are the anterior talofibular, calcaneofibular, and posterior talofibular; the major medial ligament is the deltoid. These ligaments are injured in ankle sprains with sudden inversion or eversion of the foot.

The function of the foot is to support and propel the body. The foot can adapt itself to different surfaces and absorb mechanical shocks well. The mobile medial side of the foot is more concerned with forward movement, while the lateral side of the foot functions primarily for static body support. The multiple bones of the foot are held in proper position by ligaments, muscles, and fascial bands. The plantar ligaments, primarily the spring ligament, support the arch and are supplemented in this function by the posterior tibial tendon and the plantar aponeurosis. The combination of these and other ligaments, muscles, and fascial bands provide a medial longitudinal arch. Imbalance of the muscles of the foot, as a result of neuromuscular disease or injury, causes foot deformity, because a muscle system that is usually so finely balanced cannot adapt to asymmetrical muscle activity. The intrinsic muscles of the foot include one dorsal group of short toe extensors and four layers of plantar, or sole, muscles. The first plantar layer includes adductor hallucis, flexor digitorum

brevis, and abductor digiti minimi muscles. The second group contains the lumbricals, and the third is composed of the flexor hallucis brevis, adductor hallucis, and flexor digitorum minimus brevis muscles. The fourth group is the interossei muscles. These groups are covered by the plantar fascial aponeurosis superficially. The primary bursa of the feet are the retrocalcaneal bursa, deep to the Achilles tendon, and the intercalcaneal bursa, deep to the plantar aponeurosis. Bursae that form over the head of the first metatarsal or over the lateral head of the fifth metatarsal are called bunions.

Muscles, ligaments, and fascial structures and joints must work in close conjunction to allow smooth functioning of any body movement. Any abnormality in these structures, all derived from the embryonic mesoderm, will lead to limitation in joint mobility and compromise of normal body function.

The Abdominal Wall, Inguinal Region, and Hernias

John J. White, M.D.

The abdominal wall is made up of the rectus abdominal muscles, which extend from the costal margins to the pubis on either side of the midline anteriorly, and the flat external and internal oblique and the transversus abdominis muscles lying laterally on each side. The rectus abdominis muscles are joined together by the strong fascia of the linea alba in the midline. The lateral muscles on each side originate from the costal cartilages superiorly, the lumbodorsal fascia posteriorly, and the iliac crests inferiorly. As they course anteromedially, they fuse together as a strong fascial aponeurosis, which attaches to the lateral margins of the rectus abdominis muscles. This lateral aponeurosis splits to provide both an anterior and posterior fascial sheath for the rectus abdominis muscle extending to the linea alba. In roughly the lower third, below the semilunar line of Douglas (Plate 10, dotted blue line), the aponeurotic fascia of the lateral muscles provides an anterior fascial sheath for the rectus abdominis, leaving only the endoabdominal fascia (transversalis fascia) posteriorly.

Thus, the peritoneal cavity is surrounded and shaped by a relatively strong muscular, aponeurotic, and fascial wall. Weak spots, however, may occur where muscle or fascia fail to fuse. Protrusion of an abdominal viscus through such a defect constitutes a hernia. If the viscus is not reducible back into the peritoneal cavity, it is termed an *incarcerated hernia,* and if its blood supply is compromised it is termed a *strangulated hernia.*

One area where a significant number of several kinds of hernias may develop is the groin, which compromises the inguinal and femoral canals and their contents. The inguinal canal is an oblique passage superior to the inguinal ligament (Poupart's ligament). Its entrance, the internal inguinal ring, lies just lateral to the inferior epigastric vessels, and it runs medially to the external inguinal ring, which lies over the pubic tubercle. The structures of the spermatic cord pass through the inguinal canal to the testis in the scrotum. These include the cremaster muscle and fascia, the vas deferens, the spermatic artery and veins, and the processus vaginalis. The ilioinguinal nerve lies just under the aponeurosis of the external oblique in the canal and emerges through the external ring.

The inguinal canal is the site of direct and indirect inguinal hernias. Indirect inguinal hernias occur when a viscus, usually bowel, passes through the internal ring into the canal (Plate 11, white arrow), generally via the sac of a nonobliterated processus vaginalis. The vaginal process is a peritoneal outpouching of the abdominal cavity that proceeds through the inguinal canal into the scrotum, preceding, and perhaps guiding, the descent of the testis from its retroabdominal origin to its ultimate position in the scrotum. The vaginal process remains more or less patent in approximately 25 percent of men and therefore constitutes a potential sac for herniation throughout life.

Direct inguinal hernias, on the other hand, appear to be acquired on the basis of muscular weakness in the abdominal wall. The back wall of the inguinal canal is composed only of endoabdominal fascia (the transversalis fascia) and the peritoneum. This relatively weak area constitutes the inferior part of Hesselbach's triangle, whose borders are the lateral margin of the rectus abdominis muscle medially and the inferior epigastric vessels laterally. The inguinal ligament is its base. This weak back wall of the canal, in Hesselbach's triangle, is the site of origin of direct inguinal hernias (Plate 11, green arrow).

The femoral canal lies deep to the inguinal ligament and medial to the femoral vessels. Its medial margin is the iliopectineal ridge (Cooper's ligament) and lacunar ligament; its floor is the fascia over the pectineus muscle. This canal may be the site of femoral hernias (Plate 11, pink arrow). Ordinarily it contains only fat and lymphatics that drain the leg, the groin, and the perineum.

Plate 10.
Abdominal Wall—Inguinal Region

Fifth costal cart.

Ant. rectus sheath

Ext. oblique mus.
and aponeurosis

Int. oblique
aponeurosis

Post. rectus sheath

Transversalis
fascia

Ant.-sup. iliac
spine

Ant. rectus sheath and
pyramidalis mus.

Inguinal lig.

Int. inguinal ring

Ext. inguinal ring

Lymph node of Cloquet

Reflected inguinal
lig.

Pubic tubercle

Cremaster mus.
and fascia

Dartos tunic

Scrotum

Skin

Epigastric vess.

Rectus mus.

Linea alba

Semilunar line
of Douglas

Note: Absence of post.
rectus sheath

Testicular vess.

Inf. epigastric vess.

Ext. spermatic a.

Superficial epigastric vess.

Ilioinguinal n.

Femoral canal

Femoral vess.

Fossa ovalis

Deep ext.
pudendal vess.

Parietal tunica vaginalis

Epididymis

Testis

Plate 11.
Inguinal Region

Ant. rectus sheath over rectus mus.

Int. oblique mus.

Ext. oblique mus.

Ext. oblique aponeurosis

Int. inguinal ring

Ilioinguinal n.

Inguinal lig.

Lat. cremaster mus.

Ductus deferens

Interfoveolar mus. (Hesselbach)

Beginning shelving margin of inguinal lig.

Site of Femoral Hernia Femoral Canal

Site of Indirect Hernia Internal Inguinal Ring

Int. oblique mus.

Reflected Inguinal lig.

Pubic tubercle

Inguinal falx (conjoined)

Ext. inguinal ring

Site for Relaxation Incision of Anterior Rectus Sheath during Herniorrhaphy

Transversus mus.

Hesselbach's triangle

Med. cremaster mus.

Site of Direct Hernia Transversalis Fascia (Thin Spot)

Interfoveolar lig. (Hesselbach) (Thickened transversalis) Fascia

Interfoveolar mus.

The anatomical relationship of the common varieties of hernia are shown in plate 12.

Indirect inguinal hernia is shown (upper left) in a completely patent processus vaginalis. There is dilatation of the proximal peritoneal sac within the inguinal canal due to visceral protrusion. The distal processus vaginalis in the scrotum about the testis is filled with fluid and waxes and wanes in size as the fluid leaves and enters the peritoneal cavity; this constitutes a communicating hydrocele.

A patent processus vaginalis is a more frequent occurrence than was once thought (upper right). Patency has been reported in 90 percent of neonates at autopsy and in 57 percent of babies dying before 1 year of age; an open processus vaginalis on the opposite side has been reported in 40 to 50 percent of both children and adult with unilateral inguinal hernias; and a patent processus vaginalis has been noted in 15 to 35 percent of adult autopsies. Indirect inguinal hernias in adults may occur into these open peritoneal sacs (arrow) as they do in children; in effect, they may remain as potential hernia sacs throughout life.

The distal processus vaginalis may also remain patent instead of obliterating. If the more proximal processus is obliterated, the tunica vaginalis of the testis may distend with secretions to form a noncommunicating hydrocele of the scrotum. An open area in the mid processus vaginalis can form an encysted hydrocele of the cord.

A double inguinal, or Pantaloon, hernia is shown at lower left. A typical indirect hernia emerges into the inguinal canal from the internal ring, along the same path as the patent processus vaginalis, and protrudes obliquely toward the external ring. A direct hernia is present as well, protruding through the weak back wall of the medial inguinal canal in Hesselbach's triangle. It bulges more directly toward the external ring. The interfoveolar muscle provides the support for the crotch of the pantaloons.

Some believe that most indirect hernias are congenital in nature, regardless of the age at which they occur, and that they consist of viscera entering the potential hernia sac represented by a patent processus vaginalis. Direct hernias generally appear to be acquired in nature, with peritoneal and visceral bulging through a weak point of the abdominal wall (the posterior inguinal canal).

A sliding inguinal hernia is shown at lower right. The peritoneal sac of an inguinal hernia may increase in size either by stretching of the peritoneum or by additional peritoneum sliding out of the abdominal cavity into the groin. With the latter mechanism, extraperitoneal viscera attached to the peritoneum may slide out as well. The sigmoid colon may present in this manner laterally in left-sided inguinal hernias (as pictured), or the cecum may present if the hernia is on the right side. The urinary bladder may present medially in cases of hernias on either side. Because of the sliding nature of these hernias, each of the viscera constitutes part of the respective wall of its hernia sac.

Plate 13 shows the sites of abdominal and pelvic hernias.

Hernias of the upper abdomen and diaphragm are shown in the upper left. Esophageal hiatal hernias occur through and about the esophageal hiatus of the diaphragm. This opening is most commonly formed by a decussation of the medial and lateral fibers of the right crus of the diaphragm, although it may be located within the fibers of the left crus in some instances. Two varieties of hernias about the hiatus are recognized.

The true hiatus hernia, or sliding hernia, is a displacement of the intra-abdominal portion of the esophagus, the cardiac sphincter, and perhaps the upper stomach into the chest through the hiatus. It is considered to be "sliding" because the stomach makes up part of the wall of the sac. Its symptomatology is different from that of the other types of hernias of the abdominal cavity, consisting not of incarceration and obstruction but of acid reflux, esophagitis, and possibly fibrosis.

The parahiatal hernia occurs less frequently and is a protrusion of stomach wall through the diaphragm near the hiatus, with a normally positioned esophagogastric junction. These hernias may incarcerate; esophagitis is not a problem, since the sphincter mechanism is intact.

The congenital posterolateral diaphragmatic hernia (Bochdalek's hernia) usually occurs on the left side and represents a persistently patent pleuroperitoneal canal. The diaphragm fails to form completely, and abdominal contents take residence in the chest as well. It is commonly associated with a hypoplastic lung on the side of the defect and constitutes one cause for acute respiratory distress in newborns. Treatment is directed toward reduction of the herniated abdominal viscera and repair of the defect.

The superior lumbar trigone lies beneath the latissimus dorsi muscle and is bounded superiorly by the twelfth rib, medially by the lateral margin of the paraspinous muscles (sacrospinalis), and inferiorly by the superior margin of the internal oblique muscle. Its floor is the aponeurosis of the transversus abdominis muscle. It may be the site of posterior abdominal wall hernias.

The inferior lumbar trigone (triangle of Petit) may also be the site for hernias. Its base is the iliac crest, and the floor the internal oblique muscle; the sides are the posterior margin of the external oblique and anterior border of latissimus dorsi just before they cross.

Plate 12.
Hernias

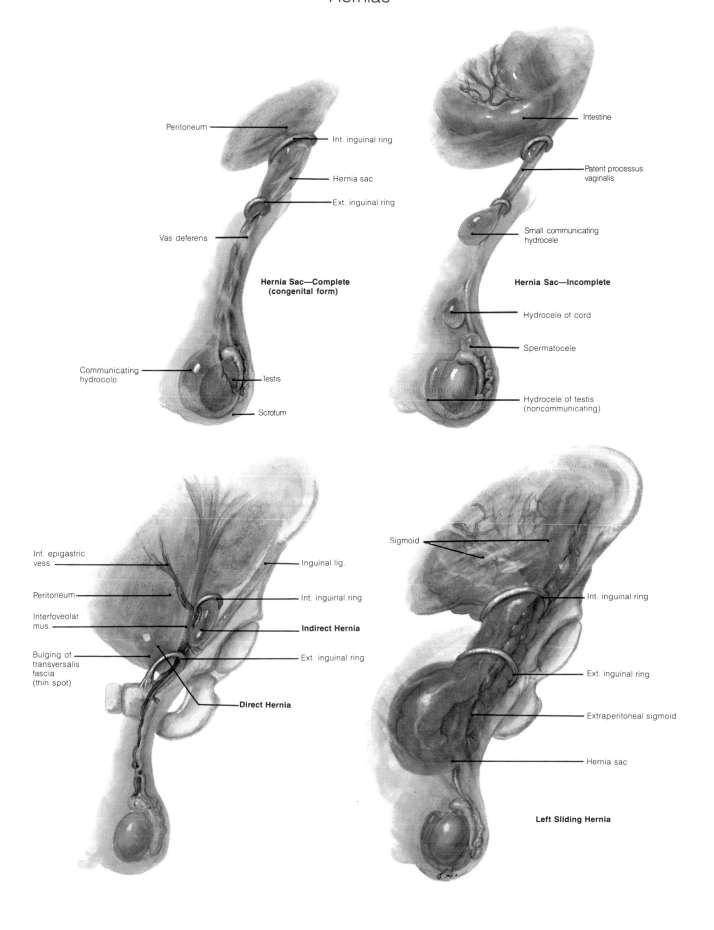

Peritoneum — Int. inguinal ring

Hernia sac

Ext. inguinal ring

Vas deferens

**Hernia Sac—Complete
(congenital form)**

Communicating hydrocolo — Testis

Scrotum

Intestine

Patent processus vaginalis

Small communicating hydrocele

Hernia Sac—Incomplete

Hydrocele of cord

Spermatocele

Hydrocele of testis (noncommunicating)

Inf. epigastric vess. — Inguinal lig.

Peritoneum — Int. inguinal ring

Interfoveolar mus. — **Indirect Hernia**

Bulging of transversalis fascia (thin spot) — Ext. inguinal ring

Direct Hernia

Sigmoid

Int. inguinal ring

Ext. inguinal ring

Extraperitoneal sigmoid

Hernia sac

Left Sliding Hernia

Plate 13.
Sites of Abdominal and Pelvic Hernias

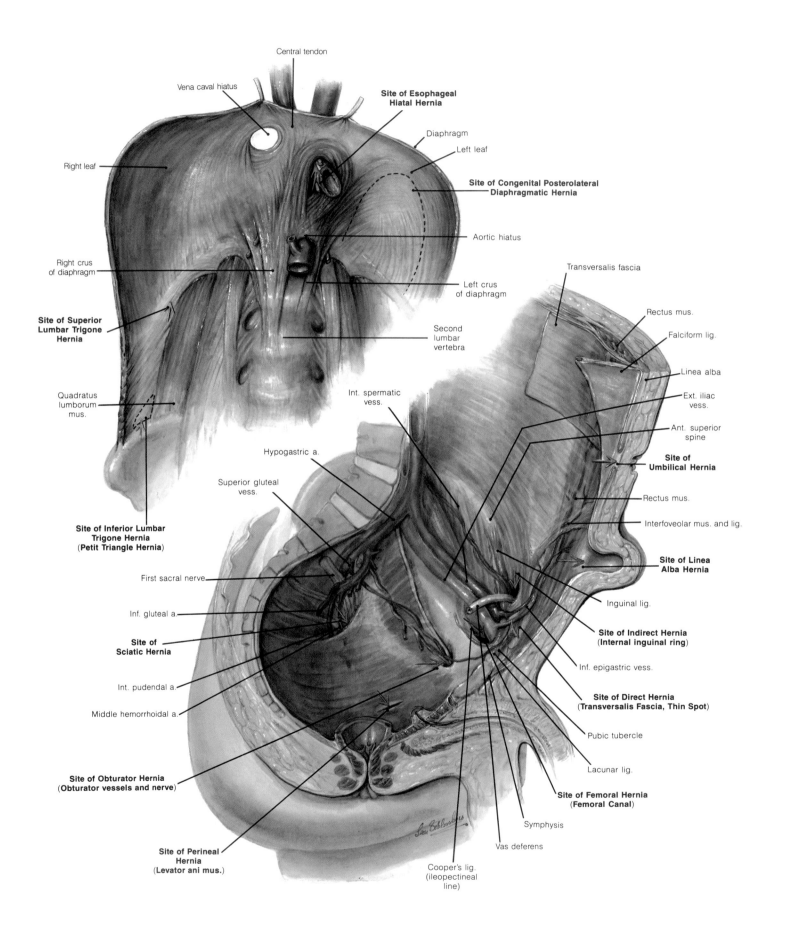

Central tendon

Vena caval hiatus

Site of Esophageal Hiatal Hernia

Diaphragm

Left leaf

Site of Congenital Posterolateral Diaphragmatic Hernia

Right leaf

Aortic hiatus

Right crus of diaphragm

Left crus of diaphragm

Transversalis fascia

Rectus mus.

Falciform lig.

Linea alba

Ext. iliac vess.

Site of Superior Lumbar Trigone Hernia

Second lumbar vertebra

Int. spermatic vess.

Ant. superior spine

Site of Umbilical Hernia

Rectus mus.

Interfoveolar mus. and lig.

Quadratus lumborum mus.

Hypogastric a.

Site of Linea Alba Hernia

Superior gluteal vess.

Site of Inferior Lumbar Trigone Hernia (Petit Triangle Hernia)

First sacral nerve

Inf. gluteal a.

Inguinal lig.

Site of Indirect Hernia (Internal inguinal ring)

Site of Sciatic Hernia

Inf. epigastric vess.

Int. pudendal a.

Site of Direct Hernia (Transversalis Fascia, Thin Spot)

Middle hemorrhoidal a.

Pubic tubercle

Site of Obturator Hernia (Obturator vessels and nerve)

Lacunar lig.

Site of Femoral Hernia (Femoral Canal)

Symphysis

Vas deferens

Site of Perineal Hernia (Levator ani mus.)

Cooper's lig. (ileopectineal line)

Hernias of the lower abdomen and pelvis are shown in the lower right. Umbilical hernias occur through a fascial defect in the linea alba at the umbilicus. This defect is usually congenital and frequently closes spontaneously. Defects larger than 1.5 cm. in diameter in children tend to remain open, and repair is usually advocated in these cases. Incarcerated umbilical hernias are rare in children, but they occur more frequently in adults, especially parous women, and are associated with significant morbidity and mortality. Repair consists of reduction of sac contents and excision of the sac with fascia-to-fascia repair of the defect.

Hernias can develop anywhere along the linea alba. Preperitoneal fat can protrude through the orifices of penetrating vessels and nerves, with great pain because of pressure on the nerves. Adjacent peritoneum may also protrude, and abdominal contents may actually herniate in the fully developed state.

There are several types of pelvic hernias that occur rather infrequently. The sciatic hernia occurs through the great sacrosciatic foramen, the oval space between the innominate bone and the lesser sacrosciatic ligament through which the sciatic nerve and inferior gluteal artery pass. Obturator hernias occur as visceral protrusions through the obturator canal, through which the obturator vessels pass. Perineal hernias develop as viscera protrude through an opening, either natural or acquired, in the levator ani muscles which comprise the pelvic diaphragm.

The Hematopoietic System and Development of Blood Cells

William R. Bell, M.D.

The hematopoietic system is composed of red blood cells, white blood cells, and platelets, and their production sites and controlling sites responsible for cellular maturation and growth (e.g., stomach, liver), plus the fluid (plasma) in which these formed elements are suspended inside blood vessels (Plate 14). In the embryo, the source of these formed elements is the connective tissue called *mesenchyme*. In the human embryo, blood cells are first formed in the blood islands of the yolk sac. At a later time, when the embryo reaches 5 to 8 mm in length, the major source of blood cells is the liver, and a few weeks later production is supplemented by sites in the thymus and spleen. By the fifth month of gestation, production sites in the liver, thymus, and spleen gradually decrease and the bone marrow takes over hematopoietic production. The fixed mesenchymal

cells are reduced to scant reticular stroma, but they remain throughout life with intact potentialities. Lymphocytes are an exception; they are produced in the lymph nodes, spleen, and thymus.

Erythropoiesis (production of red blood cells) in the infant and adult takes place continuously in the marrow of certain bones. The principal marrow sites are located in the skull, vertebrae, ribs, sternum, pelvis, femurs, and humeri. As age progresses, the vertebrae, ribs, and sternum are the major sites of hematopoietic activity. Within the bone marrow, the red cell is derived from a primitive nucleated cell called the *erythroblast*. Proliferation results from successive mitotic cell divisions (Plate 15). As maturation progresses, hemoglobin appears and the nucleus becomes smaller and is eventually extruded from the cell.

The maturation process is a complex biochemical process regulated by numerous agents. Notable among these agents is an intrinsic factor produced by the stomach. The intrinsic factor, by complexing with an extrinsic factor (vitamin B_{12}), is responsible for its absorption from the intestinal tract into the blood. The mature red cell is then introduced into the circulating blood via the vascular channels of the bone marrow. In the adult there are 0.56 gm of marrow per gram of blood, and the bone marrow approximates 3 to 6 percent of the total body weight. A steady balance between red cell production and removal of senescent red cells (more than 120 days old) from the circulation by the spleen is accurately maintained. The rate of red cell production is normally controlled by a hormone called *erythropoietin,* which is mainly produced in the kidneys.

White blood cells (leukocytes) are independently motile cells, composed of three classes, each unique and different in morphologic structure and function: granulocytes, monocytes, and lymphocytes. In general, the leukocytes survive in the circulation for two to eight days. The most numerous of the leukocytes are the granulocytes, which originate in the bone marrow and can be divided into three subtypes: neutrophils, eosinophils, and basophils. Their orderly maturation and development from precursor blasts is shown in Plate 15. They are identified by a multilobed nucleus surrounded by numerous granules in the cytoplasm. Approximately 60 to 65 percent of the leukocytes in the body are neutrophils (pink cytoplasmic granules); and the eosinophils (red cytoplasmic granules) and basophils (dark blue cytoplasmic granules) total about 3 percent. Neutrophils function is defense and repair by performing phagocytosis of foreign cells, bacteria, and other infectious organisms. Eosinophils are phagocytic and participate mainly in antigen-antibody tissue interactions. Precise information on the function of the basophil is as yet lacking.

The largest cells in the circulating blood are monocytes, which total 7 percent of all leukocytes. Their origin is probably in the bone marrow. Monocytes are motile and are capable of phagocytosis. They are identified by a large, eccentrically placed, irregular nucleus, surrounded by a variable number of pink-purple and azurophilic granules.

Lymphocytes originate in the lymph nodes, spleen, thymus, and the tonsillar and lymphoid tissue of the alimentary tract and total about 25 to 30 percent of circulating leukocytes. Lymphocytes are identified by a single circular homogeneous nucleus that occupies most of the cell and is surrounded by a rim of cytoplasm that contains very few granules. Lymphocytes function in the body as the system responsible for acquired immunity to foreign cells and antigens. One type of lymphocyte is capable of producing immunoglobulins (antibodies), and the other type is concerned with cell-mediated immunity. The latter type is responsible for rejection of transplanted organs and certain allergic reactions.

Platelets (thrombocytes) are the smallest cells in the circulating blood. Like mature red cells they lack a nucleus and are not capable of cell division. Platelets originate as segmental structures that are released into the circulation from the cytoplasm of megakaryocytes, the largest cells in the bone marrow (Plate 15). The main function of the blood platelets is participation in hemostasis, the prevention and control of bleeding. In addition, platelets function in the maintenance of the integrity of the endothelial lining of vessels. Their circulation time in the blood is about ten days.

PLASMA

Plasma is a complex solution of electrolytes, proteins (7–8 percent), and water (90 percent). The major protein is albumin, but other proteins, including antibodies, hormones, lipids, and carbohydrate-protein complexes, and the various factors and components of the coagulation system are present. The liver is the major site for the production of most of the proteins in the circulating blood. The liver is known to produce albumin, fibrinogen (Factor I), prothrombin (Factor II), and other coagulation factors that enable the blood to clot, including Factors V, VII, IX, and X. The liver also acts as a storage site for other agents that influence the production of elements in the blood. The blood produced by the hematopoietic system, the "milieu interieur," is essential for normal function and life.

Plate 14.
The Hematopoietic System

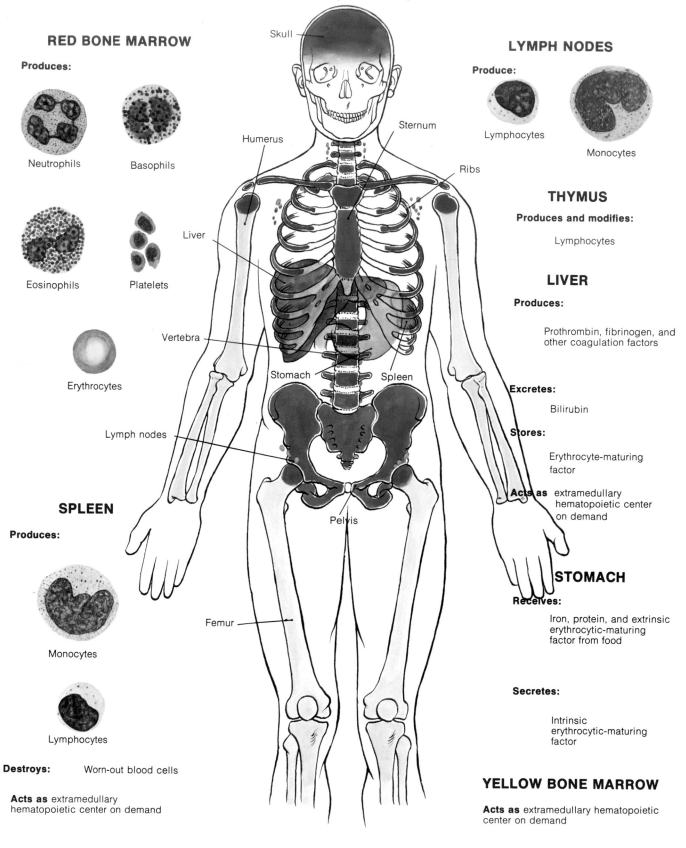

RED BONE MARROW

Produces:

Neutrophils

Basophils

Eosinophils

Platelets

Erythrocytes

SPLEEN

Produces:

Monocytes

Lymphocytes

Destroys: Worn-out blood cells

Acts as extramedullary hematopoietic center on demand

LYMPH NODES

Produce:

Lymphocytes

Monocytes

THYMUS

Produces and modifies:

Lymphocytes

LIVER

Produces:

Prothrombin, fibrinogen, and other coagulation factors

Excretes:

Bilirubin

Stores:

Erythrocyte-maturing factor

Acts as extramedullary hematopoietic center on demand

STOMACH

Receives:

Iron, protein, and extrinsic erythrocytic-maturing factor from food

Secretes:

Intrinsic erythrocytic-maturing factor

YELLOW BONE MARROW

Acts as extramedullary hematopoietic center on demand

Skull

Humerus

Sternum

Ribs

Liver

Vertebra

Stomach

Spleen

Lymph nodes

Pelvis

Femur

Plate 15.
Development of Blood Cells

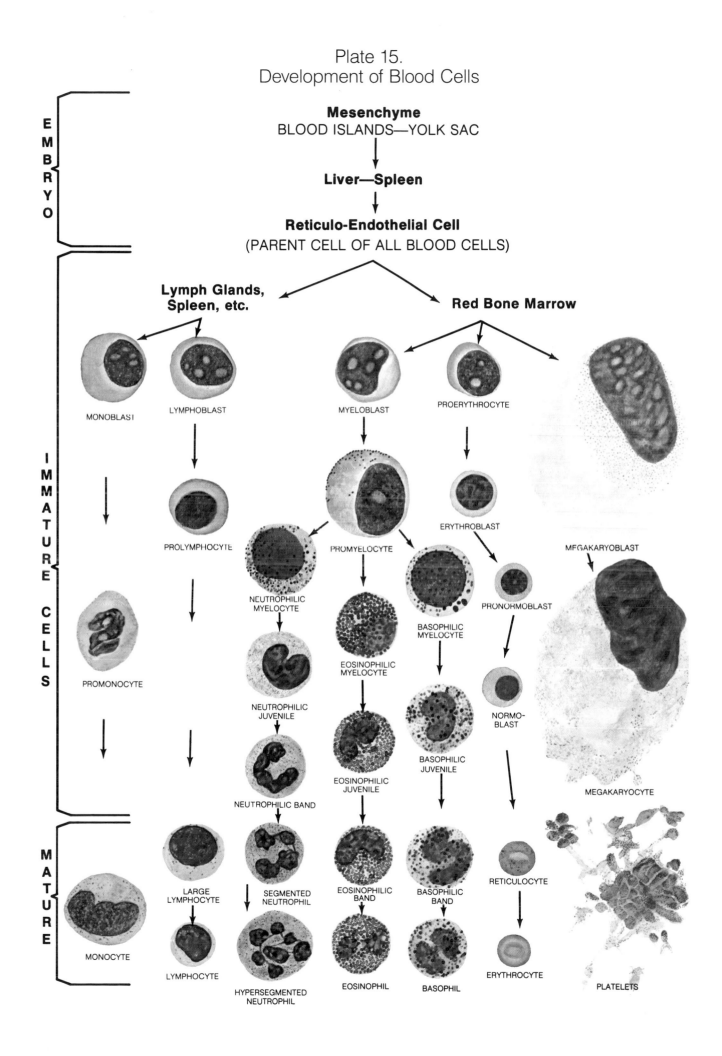

EMBRYO

Mesenchyme
BLOOD ISLANDS—YOLK SAC

Liver—Spleen

Reticulo-Endothelial Cell
(PARENT CELL OF ALL BLOOD CELLS)

Lymph Glands, Spleen, etc.

Red Bone Marrow

IMMATURE CELLS

MONOBLAST

LYMPHOBLAST

MYELOBLAST

PROERYTHROCYTE

PROLYMPHOCYTE

PROMYELOCYTE

ERYTHROBLAST

MEGAKARYOBLAST

NEUTROPHILIC MYELOCYTE

EOSINOPHILIC MYELOCYTE

BASOPHILIC MYELOCYTE

PRONORMOBLAST

PROMONOCYTE

NEUTROPHILIC JUVENILE

EOSINOPHILIC JUVENILE

BASOPHILIC JUVENILE

NORMO-BLAST

NEUTROPHILIC BAND

MEGAKARYOCYTE

MATURE

MONOCYTE

LARGE LYMPHOCYTE

SEGMENTED NEUTROPHIL

EOSINOPHILIC BAND

BASOPHILIC BAND

RETICULOCYTE

LYMPHOCYTE

HYPERSEGMENTED NEUTROPHIL

EOSINOPHIL

BASOPHIL

ERYTHROCYTE

PLATELETS

The Autonomic Nervous System

George B. Udvarhelyi, M.D.

The autonomic nervous system consists of a central and a peripheral component: information on central autonomic connections is still incomplete. A mechanism for interaction exists between the frontal cortex and the hypothalamus. The frontal cortex represents an afferent projection area that receives visceral impulses mainly from the hypothalamus, either directly or by way of the way stations in the thalamus. In response to stimulation, the frontal cortex activates other cortical areas, and issues efferent messages either directly to peripheral effectors or through the hypothalamus. Other cortical areas, like the cingulum and the posterior orbital, anterior insular, and temporal cortex, play important roles in cardiovascular function, respiratory movements, gastric motility, pupillary changes, and other autonomic responses such as piloerection, salivation, bladder contraction, and defecation. Through the cortical hypothalamic, corticothalamic, and corticostriate fibers, the different regions of the cerebral cortex are connected with the second important structure of the central part of the autonomic system, namely, the hypothalamus. Stimulation of various areas of the hypothalamus evokes special responses. Excitation of the anterior hypothalamic region produces bladder contraction, increase of gastrointestinal mobility, cardiac depression, and vasodilatation. Drowsiness, unconsciousness, and slowing of the heart occur in man after stimulation of the preoptic area. Excitation of the posterior and lateral regions of the hypothalamus results in the elevation of blood pressure, cardiac acceleration, pupillary dilatation, sweating, piloerection, hypoglycemia, and arrest of gastrointestinal movements. In animals, these effects are usually accompanied by expression of fear and rage. Control of body temperature is achieved in warm-blooded animals by release of excess heat through peripheral vasodilatation, sweating, and panting. Hunger and thirst are regulated by the hypothalamus, the appetite being inhibited by the ventromedial part, whereas the lateral and posterior hypothalamic regions seem to promote it. Stimulation of the dorsal hypothalamus increases the urge for drinking, whereas lesions of the hypothalamus result in hypodipsia. Observation in experimental animals and humans confirms that the anterior region of the hypothalamus is primarily concerned with the regulation of parasympathetic activities, whereas the posterior and lateral hypothalamic areas govern sympathetic responses. The pituitary gland is partly under the influence of the hypothalamus and partly controlled by a feedback mechanism of other endocrine glands. Through the anterior lobe of the pituitary gland, the hypothalamus participates in the control of the sex cycle, the activity of the adrenal cortex, and the function of the thyroid gland. Through the neuroendocrine connections to the posterior pituitary lobe, the hypothalamus controls the production of antidiuretic hormone and also the release of oxytocin.

The peripheral component of the autonomic nervous system consists of an efferent motor and an afferent sensory division. The peripheral motor autonomic division consists of two neurons: a preganglionic one, which has its cell of origin in the central nervous system, which synapses with several cell bodies of the second, the postganglionic neurons. The postganglionic nerve fibers terminate at the effectors, i.e., smooth muscle, glands, and heart. Preganglionic nerve fibers are covered with a thin myelin sheet and are white when viewed in the fresh state. Preganglionic neurons manufacture a chemical substance, acetylcholine, and are therefore called *cholinergic*. Postganglionic nerve fibers are unmyelinated and therefore are gray in appearance. Some postganglionic fibers are cholinergic, but the majority produce an adrenalinelike or noradrenalinelike substance for the stimulation of the effectors and are therefore called *adrenergic*.

According to the striking differences in the anatomical arrangement and functional significance, the motor autonomic nerves have been divided into two components, the parasympathetic division (craniosacral) and the sympathetic (thoracolumbar) outflow of the autonomic nervous system. The preganglionic parasympathetic nerve fibers leave the central nervous system at four places:

1. Hypothalamic outflow.

2. Tectal outflow. Preganglionic fibers originate from the Edinger-Westphal nucleus traveling along the third cranial nerve and terminate at the ciliary ganglion. The postganglionic fibers supply the sphincter of the pupil and the ciliary muscles. Stimulation produces contraction of the pupil and accommodation to near and far vision.

3. Bulbar outflow. Parasympathetic fibers arise from the nuclei of the rhombencephalon to innervate the salivary glands and the viscera in the thorax and abdomen. Preganglionic fibers travel along the facial nerve, with postganglionic participation in the lacrimal glands, and in the sphenopalatine, submaxillary, and sublingual glands. Stimulation produces increased secretion. The outflow of autonomic fibers along the facial nerve contains vasodilator nerve fibers for the middle meningeal arteries and vasomotor fibers for the blood vessels of the face. The glossopharyngeal nerve carries fibers to the parotid gland. The dorsal vagus nucleus is the origin of preganglionic fibers, with postganglionic release within the auricles of the heart and in the mesenteric plexuses of the intestinal wall. The vagal nerve fibers slow the heart, constrict the smooth muscle in the small bronchi of the lung, increase the activity of the pancreas and liver, and, except for the sphincter muscles of these regions, promote peristalsis of the stomach and intestine.

4. Sacral outflow. The preganglionic fibers arising from the lateral gray matter of the spinal cord travel with the ventrospinal nerve roots of the midsacral region into the pelvis. After synapsis in postganglionic cell bodies that are placed in the pelvic plexuses and in the walls of the bladder and rectum, the fibers terminate at the lower segment of the colon, the rectum, the bladder, and the genital system. Stimulation will produce contraction of the smooth muscles of the bladder and rectum and relaxation of the internal sphincters, resulting in emptying of the bladder and rectum.

The sympathetic division or the thoracolumbar outflow of the autonomic nervous system consists of short preganglionic neurons, which terminate with many collaterals at postganglionic cell bodies. The cell bodies of the postganglionic neurons, which have longer fibers, are remote from their organs of supply. They form conspicuous ganglia, which are placed along the side and in front of the spine, enabling sympathetic discharges to spread widely throughout the body, whereas parasympathetic impulses remain confined to more limited areas. The preganglionic sympathetic neurons are cholinergic, but the postganglionic sympathetic neurons by and large are adrenergic. The finely myelinated preganglionic fibers arising from the spinal cord travel along the ventral spinal roots of the thoracic and upper lumbar spinal nerves. Just beyond the intervertebral foramen, these fibers leave each of the spinal nerves as a white ramus communicans, which enters its corresponding paravertebral ganglion, which is present at each segment lateral to and along the entire length of the spine. Other portions of preganglionic fibers pass through and run as splanchnic nerves to the synaptic junctions in the prevertebral ganglia, such as the celiac, superior, and inferior mesenteric ganglia, which are placed in front of the spine. The unmyelinated postganglionic fibers arise from the paravertebral ganglion and join as gray rami communicantes the spinal nerves in which they travel to the blood vessels, sweat glands, and erector pilorum muscles of the skin, and probably also to the blood vessels of the striated muscles and bone. Stimulation will produce constriction of the blood vessels, increased sweating (hyperhidrosis), and piloerection. The regulation of body temperature is achieved by hyperactivity of the sweat glands and vasodilatation as response to heat, and by vasoconstriction and decreased sweat activity as response to cold, mediated through the sympathetic fibers alone. The term *sympathetic trunk* was coined to describe the chain or cord that extends from the base of the skull to the lower end of the spine.

The majority of afferent impulses from the viscera of the peritoneal cavity are transmitted by fibers of the sympathetic nervous system. These afferent fibers arise from the viscera and travel with the arteries of the viscera to reach a series of plexuses which are located around the major branches of the abdominal aorta. They traverse these plexuses without synapsis and become the splanchnic nerves. The afferent fibers subsequently enter the ganglia of the sympathetic chain which they again traverse without synapsis to enter the spinal cord via the white rami. Within the spinal cord, the impulses traversing the viscerosensory nerve fibers stimulate the somatic sensory nerve fibers arising from the same level of the cord and innervating various dermatomes of the abdominal wall. Pain arising from an intra-

Plate 16.
Autonomic Nervous System and Effects of Stimulation (Respiratory and Digestive Systems

Maintains Activity of Involuntary Visceral Effectors

(Organs below Level of Consciousness)

EFFECTS OF STIMULATION
RESPIRATORY AND DIGESTIVE SYSTEMS

The hypothalamic nuclei and vasomotor and respiratory centers are principal sites for correlation and integration of impulses from cortex, visceral organs, and/or hormones in blood. Translate stimuli into physiological activity to maintain functional equilibrium.

Sympathetic

Parietal lobe
Premotor area
Hypothalamic nuclei
Frontal lobe
Occipital lobe
Temporal lobe
Respiratory center
Vasomotor center
(Pons medulla oblongata)
Int. carotid n.
Ext. carotid n.
Sup. cervical gang.
Middle cervical gang.
Stellate gang.
Cardiac plexus
Pulmonary plexus
Sympathetic chain
White ramus communicans
Greater splanchnic nn. T5–9
Lesser splanchnic nn. T10–11
Celiac gang.
Aorticorenal gang.
To kidney, ureter, ovary, and testis
Least splanchnic n.
Renal plexus
To genitourinary system
Sup. mesenteric plexus
Inf. mesenteric plexus
Sup. hypogastric plexus
Hypogastric n.
Pelvic plexus
To ureter, bladder, prostate, uterus, fallop. tube, vagina, and ext. genitalia

Cervical nn. 1–8
Thoracic nn. 1–12
Thoracolumbar sympathetic outflow T1–L3
Lumbar nn. 1–5
Sacral nn. 1–5
Coccygeal n.

Sympathetic stimulation

Bronchodilatation— inhibits bronchial glandular secretion

Stimulates slight output of thick mucus secretions from salivary glands; inhibition of peristalsis, tone, and secretions of esoph., stomach, and intestines; contraction of sphincters; relaxes gallbladder and ducts

Dilatation of pupil

Ciliary gang.
Pupillary sphincter and ciliary mus.
Lacrimal gland
To heart

Parasympathetic stimulation

Bronchoconstriction— stimulates bronchial glandular secretion

Stimulation of copious thin watery secretions from salivary glands; stimulation of peristalsis, tone, and secretions of esoph., stomach, and intestines; relaxation of sphincters; contraction of gallbladder and ducts

Contraction of pupillary sphincter and contraction of ciliary mus.

Salivary glands (parotid, submandibular, and sublingual)

Parasympathetic

Hypothalamic nuclei
Oculomotor n.
Facial n.
Cranial outflow
Glossopharyngeal n.
Vagus n.
Otic gang.
Sphenopalatine gang.
Ciliary gang.
Submandibular gang.
Cardiac plexus
Celiac plexus
Pulmonary plexus
Pelvic plexus
Rectum
To kidney, ureter, bladder, ovary, testis, and ext. genitalia

Key:
Ganglion and synapse
Preganglionic fiber (cholinergic)
Postganglionic fiber (adrenergic)

Postganglionic motor fibers via gray rami communicans to spinal n. and the cephalic portion of the sympathetic system for distribution to blood vess., sweat glands, and piloerector mus. of hairs

Key:
Ganglion and synapse
Postganglionic fiber (cholinergic)
Preganglionic fiber (cholinergic)

Plate 17.
Autonomic Nervous System—Mechanism of Effector Organ Stimulation (Neurohormonal and Genitourinary Systems)

Parietal lobe

Hypothalamus

Occipital lobe

Frontal lobe

Impulses from cerebral centers descend in spinal cord and nerve fibers to effector organs.

Temporal lobe

Vasomotor center

Respiratory center

Sympathetic stimulation

Mainly adrenergic, releases epinephrine and/or norepinephrine at nerve ending.

Sympathetic fibers

Smooth muscle

Contraction of cells

Vena cava

Relaxation of cells

Muscular exertion, emotional stimulation, rage, fright (alarm reflex) stimulate release of epinephrine and norepinephrine from adrenal medulla into bloodstream. Effector cells are reached throughout entire body via circulation to augment or inhibit activity of effector organs.

Release of epinephrine or norepinephrine at nerve ending (myoneural junction) causes contraction or relaxation of cells (vasoconstriction, vasodilatation, glandular activity, peristalsis, etc.).

Parasympathetic stimulation

Mainly cholinergic, releases acetylcholine at nerve ending

Parasympathetic fibers

Smooth muscle

Relaxation of cells

Contraction of cells

Release of acetylcholine at nerve ending (myoneural junction) causes relaxation or contraction of cells, augments glandular secretions, stimulates peristalsis, etc.

EFFECTS OF STIMULATION
NEUROHORMONAL AND GENITOURINARY SYSTEMS

Sympathetic stimulation

Constricts vessels of kidneys; decreases tone of ureter and relaxes bladder muscle; contracts trigonal and sphincter muscles; stimulates sex organs

Parasympathetic stimulation

Increases tone of ureter and contracts bladder muscle; relaxes trigonal and sphincter muscles; depresses sex organs

Vena cava

Adrenal medulla

Celiac gang.

Pelvic plexus

Inf. mesenteric plexus

Kidneys

Ureters

Bladder

Pelvic plexus

Pelvic n.

Regulation of Body Temperature

Sympathetic stimulation

Hyperactivity of sweat glands

Vasoconstriction of blood vessels of skin

Sweat

Parasympathetic stimulation

None

Response to heat

Decreased activity of sweat glands

Vasodilatation of blood vessels of skin

Response to cold

Plate 18.
Visceral Afferent Pathways and Referred Areas of Pain

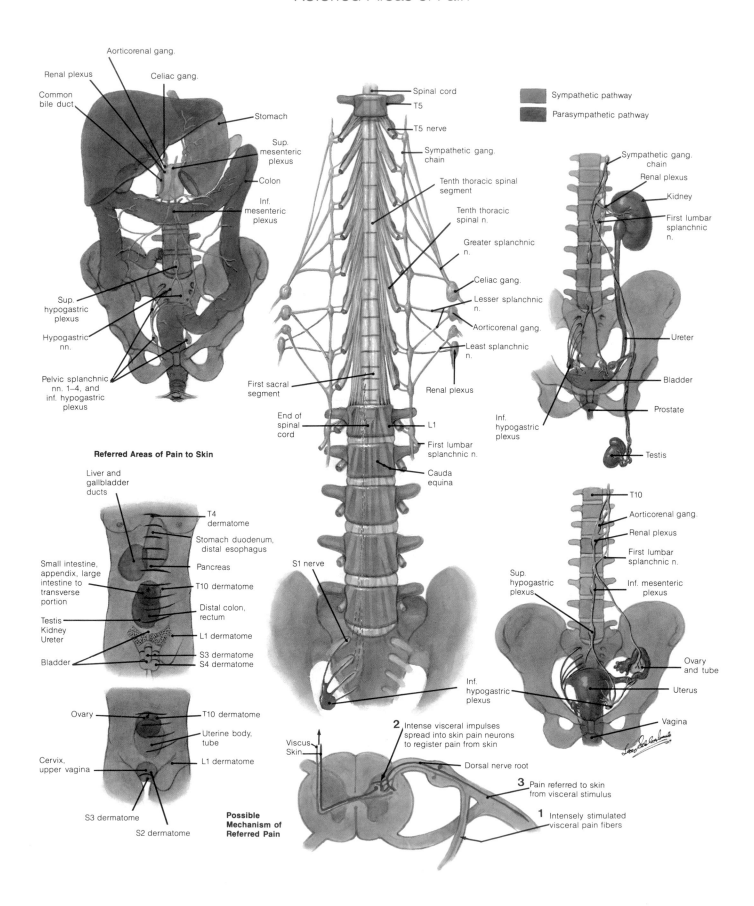

Aorticorenal gang.

Renal plexus

Celiac gang.

Common bile duct

Stomach

Sup. mesenteric plexus

Colon

Inf. mesenteric plexus

Sup. hypogastric plexus

Hypogastric nn.

Pelvic splanchnic nn. 1–4, and inf. hypogastric plexus

Spinal cord

T5

T5 nerve

Sympathetic gang. chain

Tenth thoracic spinal segment

Tenth thoracic spinal n.

Greater splanchnic n.

Celiac gang.

Lesser splanchnic n.

Aorticorenal gang.

Least splanchnic n.

Renal plexus

First sacral segment

End of spinal cord

L1

First lumbar splanchnic n.

Cauda equina

S1 nerve

Inf. hypogastric plexus

Sympathetic pathway

Parasympathetic pathway

Sympathetic gang. chain

Renal plexus

Kidney

First lumbar splanchnic n.

Ureter

Bladder

Prostate

Inf. hypogastric plexus

Testis

T10

Aorticorenal gang.

Renal plexus

First lumbar splanchnic n.

Inf. mesenteric plexus

Sup. hypogastric plexus

Ovary and tube

Uterus

Vagina

Referred Areas of Pain to Skin

Liver and gallbladder ducts

T4 dermatome

Stomach duodenum, distal esophagus

Pancreas

Small intestine, appendix, large intestine to transverse portion

T10 dermatome

Distal colon, rectum

Testis Kidney Ureter

L1 dermatome

Bladder

S3 dermatome
S4 dermatome

Ovary

T10 dermatome

Uterine body, tube

Cervix, upper vagina

L1 dermatome

S3 dermatome

S2 dermatome

Possible Mechanism of Referred Pain

Viscus
Skin

2 Intense visceral impulses spread into skin pain neurons to register pain from skin

Dorsal nerve root

3 Pain referred to skin from visceral stimulus

1 Intensely stimulated visceral pain fibers

peritoneal viscus is therefore not localized to the involved organ but rather to the dermatome supplied by the peripheral nerve entering the cord at the same levels as the viscerosensory nerve fibers.

The celiac plexus is the largest of the autonomic plexuses and surrounds the celiac arterial trunk. The celiac plexus is connected to the thoracic sympathetic trunk via the greater, lesser, and least splanchnic nerves. The greater splanchnic nerves enter the spinal cord from T5 through T9, the lesser splanchnic nerves enter from T10 to T11, and the least splanchnic nerves enter the spinal cord at T12. The celiac plexus transmits afferent sensory fibers from the stomach, liver, gallbladder, and pancreas which reach the spinal cord through the greater splanchnic nerve via the thoracic sympathetic chain. In addition, the celiac plexus also transmits afferent sensory fibers from the kidney, upper ureter, testis, and ovary which reach the spinal cord through the lesser splanchnic nerves via the thoracic sympathetic chain.

The superior mesenteric plexus receives afferent sensory nerves from the duodenum, entire small bowel, and proximal large bowel to the distal transverse colon. This plexus surrounds the origin of the superior mesenteric artery and is a continuation of the lower portion of the celiac plexus. The sensory nerves traverse this plexus without synapsis and travel via the lesser splanchnic nerves through the thoracic sympathetic chain to enter the spinal cord between T10 and T11.

The inferior mesenteric plexus is located around the origin of the inferior mesenteric artery and receives pain impulses from the distal part of the transverse and sigmoid colon. The impulses traverse this plexus, again without synapsis, and reach the lower thoracic and lumbar sympathetic chains via the least and first lumbar splanchnic nerves and enter the cord at T11, T12, and L1.

The superior and inferior hypogastric plexuses receive afferent sensory nerves from the pelvic organs and are located adjacent to the abdominal aorta and on either side of the pelvic viscera. They are joined to each other by the hypogastric nerves. Sensory fibers from the rectum, distal ureter, dome of the bladder, fundus of the uterus, and fallopian tubes traverse these plexuses and reach the spinal cord at the T11, T12, and L1 levels by traveling through the first lumbar splanchnic nerves and the higher lumbar and lower thoracic sympathetic chains. Pain impulses from the bladder neck, prostate, distal rectum, uterine cervix, and upper vagina are connected to the spinal cord through the inferior hypogastric plexus via the *parasympathetic pelvic splanchnic nerves* which enter the cord at the S2, S3, and S4 levels.

Painful stimuli, which give rise to impulses that pass along these afferent sympathetic and parasympathetic nerves, are triggered by three mechanisms: (1) an increase in intraluminal pressure of a hollow viscus; (2) ischemia of a viscus; or (3) the stretching of the capsule of a solid organ such as the liver, spleen, and kidney.

Abdominal pain can be divided into two phases. Changes in the character of the pain from one phase to the next indicates a progression of the disease process within the abdomen. The first phase of abdominal pain is called true visceral pain. It results from the distention of a viscus usually secondary to spasm of smooth muscle. Visceral pain is characterized as an ache that is not sharp or localized but diffuse and vague and generally referred to the midline. This pain is not associated with muscle rigidity or voluntary guarding of the abdominal muscles. The second phase of abdominal pain is called referred pain. This pain is due to continued stimulation of visceral pain fibers and subsequent involvement of both the visceral and somatic sensory nerve pathways. As a result of the crossover stimulation between the viscerosensory fibers and the sensory fibers of the somatic nerves, the pain is referred to the superficial area of the body surface or dermatome supplied by the peripheral somatic nerve arising from the same segment of the cord. This pain occurs when the irritable focus within a viscus has increased, giving rise to stronger stimuli, and usually indicates some type of pathology within the viscus. The pain, because of its relationship to the somatic dermatome, is fairly well localized to specific areas of the abdominal wall. This pain is usually associated with muscle guarding but not true rigidity.

It is important to appreciate the significance of these referred pain patterns, since they almost invariably indicate the presence of pathology within the abdominal cavity. Pain from the stomach and duodenum is referred to the epigastric area. Painful stimuli from the liver, gallbladder, and bowel ducts are localized to the right midepigastrium. Inflammation of the pancreas gives rise to referred pain in the epigastrium as well as directly through to the back. Pain from the small intestines is referred to the paraumbilical area. Pain from the appendix and large intestines up to the transverse colon is also referred to the paraumbilical area. Pain from the distal portion of the colon down to the upper rectum is referred to the suprapubic region. Pain from the kidney, upper ureter, ovary, and testicle is referred to the low epigastrium, paraumbilical, and flank areas. Bladder pain is referred to the suprapubic areas as well as the tip of the penis in males. Pain from the uterus, fallopian tubes, and ovaries is referred to the suprapubic area.

The physiological significance of the autonomic nervous system has been summarized by Pick in the following way: The parasympathetic or cranial sacral component is essentially an anabolic system, because it is directed toward the preservation, accumulation, and storage of energies in the body. In contrast, the general effect of the sympathetic nervous system is catabolic because it causes the expenditure of bodily energies and inhibits the intake and assimilation of nutrient matter. There is, therefore, a high degree of stability of bodily function under the dual control of the autonomic nervous system. However, the importance of ability of the body to cope with extremely difficult environmental conditions has been stressed and formulated by Cannon, who suggested a special designation, *homeostasis,* for the highly sophisticated coordination of physiological processes that maintain most of the steady states in the organism.

The Peripheral Nerves

George B. Udvarhelyi, M.D.

The peripheral nervous system consists of thirty-one pairs of segmentally arranged spinal nerves that connect the spinal cord with the various parts of the body. There are eight cervical, twelve thoracic, five lumbar, five sacral, and usually one coccygeal spinal nerve. The first cervical nerve emerges between the occipital bone and the atlas; the eight cervical nerves emerge between the seven cervical and the first thoracic vertebrae; and below that, each spinal nerve emerges from the intervertebral foramen between its own and the next lower vertebra. Each spinal nerve has a posterior and an anterior (dorsal) afferent and ventral (efferent) root. At the level of the intervertebral foramen, the posterior root forms the spinal ganglion, which contains the central origin of the afferent fibers. The ventral root does not have a ganglion but joins the posterior root, and both emerge from the intervertebral foramen as a mixed spinal nerve. This common nerve trunk contains both afferent and efferent fibers. The ventral roots, with the exception of the cervical roots, contain efferent fibers of the sympathetic nervous system.

Shortly after the spinal nerves have been formed by the union of the two roots, they divide into ventral and dorsal primary divisions. The dorsal primary division splits into branches, which supply the dorsal-axial musculature and adjacent skin. The ventral primary divisions, with the exception of those in the thoracic region, form four main plexuses: cervical, brachial, lumbar, and sacral. Those in the thoracic region, except the first, remain separate and divide individually into branches that supply the muscles and skin of the thoracic and abdominal walls. In the formation of the four main plexuses, the nerve fibers rearrange themselves into peripheral nerves. In addition to the motor and sensory impulses carried by the posterior and anterior roots, the sympathetic nervous system participates as well, this participation consisting of visceral efferent and visceral afferent fibers, which control the vasomotor, visceral, and sweat gland function throughout the somatic areas.

From the anatomical description it is clear that almost all peripheral nerves are mixed nerves containing: (1) efferent or motor fibers, (2) afferent or sensory fibers, and (3) postganglionic fibers of the sympathetic nervous system. Most peripheral nerves are composed of fibers of three or more spinal segments. Certain cranial nerves (III, VII, IX, and X) and the sacral nerves of the second, third, and fourth segments contain preganglionic fibers of the parasympathetic autonomic nervous system.

Because peripheral nerves are mixed nerves, some anatomic principles should be emphasized that have considerable clinical importance. In terms of the motor component of the peripheral nerve, there is distinction between a radicular paralysis and a peripheral nerve paralysis. If there is paralysis of a group of muscles, each supplied by the same peripheral nerve, the site of the lesion must be peripheral. On the other hand, if there is paralysis of a group of muscles each of which has the same radicular innervation, the lesion must be located in the anterior roots or spinal cord.

The cervical plexus (C1–C4) innervates the deep cervical muscles, serving the function of flexion, extension, and rotation of the neck. The cervical nerves also innervate the scalene muscles, and the phrenic nerve the diaphragm, both serving inspiration.

The sensory branches supply the skin of the lateral occipital portion of the scalp, the upper median part of the auricle, and the area over the mastoid process innervated by the small occipital nerve (C2–3); the skin of the back of the ear and over the front of the neck by the cervical cutaneous nerves (C2–3). The supraclavicular branches (C3–4) supply the skin over the clavicle and upper deltoid and pectoral regions as low as the third rib.

Irritative lesions like meningitis or high spinal cord tumors are occasionally responsible for symptoms of a cervico-occipital neuralgia; peripheral lesions are relatively rare in the cervical region because of the protection afforded by the surrounding muscles.

The brachial plexus (C5–T1) is formed by the anterior primary divisions of the last four cervical and first thoracic nerves. The relationship of the brachial plexus with the cervical-thoracic vertebral column, with the first rib, with Sibson's fascia, and with the three scalenus muscles plays an important part of the functional anatomy of this structure. As Plates 19 and 20 show, both the relationship of the plexus to these structures and also the various clinical symptoms can be better understood if one grasps the organization within the plexus itself. The brachial plexus is composed of three different components:

The roots of the plexus: C5–C6 fuse to form the upper trunk; C7 becomes the middle trunk and C8 and T1 fuse to form the lower trunk.

The middle portion of the plexus is formed by three trunks; each divides into anterior and posterior divisions. The lateral cord is formed by the anterior divisions of the upper and middle trunks; the medial cord is formed by the anterior division of the lower trunk, and the posterior cord is formed by the three posterior divisions of the upper, middle, and lower trunk. Finally, the three cords, lateral, posterior, and medial, split to form the main branches of the plexus. The position of the cords is in relation to the axillary artery. Branches from the medial and lateral cords form the median nerve; the rest of the lateral cord becomes the musculocutaneous nerve. Another portion of the medial cord forms the ulnar nerve; and the posterior cord divides to become the radial and axillary nerves. Compression by an anomalous cervical rib, by the first rib, and by the scaleni muscles will give rise to well-defined clinical symptomatology.

Numerous smaller nerves arise from the roots of the plexus; the posterior thoracic nerves (dorsal scapular nerve) (C5), the long thoracic nerve (of Bell) (C5–6–7), and rami to the scaleni and longus colli muscles. Several branches arise from the trunks: to the subclavius muscle and to the supra- and infraspinatus muscles by the suprascapular nerve. Several branches from the cords supply the pectoralis major and minor muscles through the medial and lateral anterior thoracic nerves; the upper subscapular nerve from the posterior cord innervates the subscapularis muscle (C5–6); the latissimus dorsi muscle is innervated by the middle (long) subscapular and thoracodorsal nerves (C7–8); and the lower subscapular nerve (C5–6) innervates the teres major and part of the subscapularis muscle. It should be mentioned that from the medial cord (C8–T1) sensory branches go to the medial surface of the forearm (medial antebrachial cutaneous nerve) and to the medial surface of the arm (medial brachial cutaneous nerve). The main branches of the brachial plexus are the musculocutaneous nerve (C4–5–6), the median nerve (C5–6–7–8 and T1), and the ulnar nerve (C8, T1). Nerves from the plexus trunks and partly from the cord innervate the muscles servicing the movements of the scapula, elevation, rotation, abduction, and depression of the arm.

The musculocutaneous nerve innervates the biceps and coracobrachialis and brachialis muscles and controls flexion and supination of the forearm and elevation and abduction of the arm. The median nerve innervates the flexors of the hand and fingers (except the flexor carpi ulnaris and the ulnar half of the flexor digitorum profundus) and the pronators serving the flexion of the hand and fingers and pronation. It may be compressed by the thickened transverse ligament (Plate 20). The ulnar nerve innervates the ulnar flexor muscles, the adductor pollicis, hypothenar muscles, and third and fourth lumbricales and the interossei muscles, serving the movements of the little finger, flexion of the first phalanx and extension of the other phalanges of the fourth and fifth fingers, and the spreading apart and bringing together of the fingers. Its superficial location in the olecranon groove may give rise to dysfunction of compression, requiring a surgical transposition. The radial nerve provides the innervation of the triceps, brachioradialis, and extensor muscles of the fingers, serving extension, partial flexion, and supination of the forearm, hand, and fingers. The thoracic nerves innervate the thoracic and abdominal muscles, serving elevation of the ribs (expiration and abdominal compression).

The lumbar plexus is located in the substance of the psoas muscle and is the upper portion of the lumbosacral plexus. There are five pairs of lumbar nerves; the anterior primary divisions of the first three, part of the fourth, and in 50 percent of the population part of the twelfth thoracic nerve, contribute to the lumbar plexus. Most of the branches of the lumbar plexus, which derive from the upper lumbar nerves, innervate the skin: the iliohypogastric nerve (T12, L1), the upper lateral part of the thigh and the symphysis; the ilioinguinal (L1), the upper medial part of the thigh and the root of the penis and scrotum; the genitofemoral nerve (L1–2), the scrotum and labia; the lateral femoral cutaneous nerve (L2–L3), the anterolateral side of the thigh. This nerve is responsible for unpleasant paresthesias (meralgia parasthetica) if it is strangulated or partially damaged.

The lumbar plexus (T12–L4) gives rise to the femoral nerve (iliopsoas, sartorius, and quadriceps muscles) and to the obturator nerve (the adductors of the thigh, gracilis, and external obturator muscles), serving flexion of the hip and upper and lower

Plate 19.
Peripheral Nerves
(Exclusive of Cranial Nerves)

Trigeminal
Gr. auricular
Cerv. cutan.
Brachial plex.

Cervical plex. C1–C4
Brachial plex. C5–T1
Post. cord
Lat. cord
Med. cord
Musculocutan.
Spinal cord
Median
Ulnar
Phrenic and lower thoracic innervate diaphragm
Iliohypogast.
Ilioinguin.
Radial
Genitofemoral
Lat. femoral cutaneous
Lumbosacral cord
Pudendal plex. S1–S5 and C1
Obturator
Digital branches
Femoral

T1
Intercostal nn.

Pectoralis major
Ant. serratus

Pronator radii teres
Supinator longus
Ext. carp. rad. longus
Ext. carp. rad. brev.
Flexor carpi radialis
Ext. of thumb
Ext. com. digitorum

C6–8 cerv.

Lumbar plex.
Sacral plex. L4–S3
Sup. gluteal
Inf. gluteal
Coccygeal plex. S3–C
Sciatic
Post. femoral cutan.

Pudendal
Saphenous

Sternomastoid
Scalene
Trapez.
Deltoid
Triceps
Biceps
Rectus abdominis
Oblique 8–12 intercostal–L1
Iliopsoas
Pectineus
Add. longus
Rectus femoris
Gracilis
Sartorius
Vastus interm.

Cervical plex.
T7–L1 intercostal
Lumbar plex.

Biceps
Triceps   (cerv. plex.)
Deltoid
Teres
Infraspinatus
Rhomboid
Latissimus dorsi
Sacrospinalis → All spinal
Gluteus medius
Gluteus maximus
Tensor fasciae latae

Brachial plex.
Sacral plex.

Splenius
Cervical plex.
Trapezius

Com. peroneal
Lat. cutan. sural
Med. cutan. sural
Deep peroneal
Sup. peroneal

Gr. occip.
Less. occip.
Less. occip. and gr. auric.
Supraclavic.
Axillary
Med. br. thor.
Lat. antibrach. cutan.
Lat. br. thor.
Intercosto-brach.
T12
L1
Med. brach. cutan.
Radial
Ulnar
Dor. antibrach. cutan.
Median
Post. div. L1, 2, 3
Med. antibr. cutan.
Post. div. S1, 2, 3
Lat. fem. cutan.
Lat. plantar
Ant. fem. cutan.
Sural
Med. plantar
Post. fem. cutan.
Tibial
Saphenous
Lat. plantar
Com. peroneal
Sural
Sup. peroneal
Med. plantar

Tibial
Med. cutan. sural

Peripheral sensory cutan. distribution

Ophthalmic
Maxillary
Mandibular
Gr. auric.
Supraclavic.
Axillary
Dorsal antibrach. cutan.
Cerv. cutan.
Med. br. thor.
Med. brach. cutan.
Lat. br. thor.
Med. antibr. cutan.
Sup. br. radial
Lumboing.
Lat. anti-brach. cutan.
Lat. fem. cutan.
Median
Com. peroneal
Intercostobrach.
Saphenous
Ulnar
Sup. peroneal
Deep peroneal
Ant. fem. cutan.
Med. and lat. plantar

(Cranial)
C2 C3
C3   C4 C5
C4   T1
C5   C6
T1   C7
T2   T12
C6   L1
C7   L5
C8   S1
S3   S2
S4   C8
        L5
L4   L3
        S1
        L5
L4

Radicular sensory cutan. (dermatomes) distribution

Plate 20.
Peripheral Nerves, Including Cervical, Brachial, and Lumbosacral Plexuses

Cervical plexus C1–C4
- 1st cerv. n.
- 1st cerv. vert.
- C4 n.
- C5 n.

Brachial plexus C5–T1
- 1st thor. n.

Post. cord
Clavicle
Lat. cord
Musculocutaneous n.

C4 vert.
Phrenic n.
Ant. scalenus mus.
Middle scalenus mus.
Post. scalenus mus.
Clavicle
Subclavian a.
Subclavian v.
1st rib
2nd rib
Subclavian a.
Axillary a.

Med. cord
Long thoracic n.
Thoracodorsal n.
Ulnar n.
Median n.
Medial epicondyle of humerus

Tendon biceps brachii
Lacertus fibrosus
Radial n. superf. and deep br.
Flexor carpi radialis mus.
Radial n. and a.
Common interosseous a.
Dorsal interosseous a.
Volar interosseous a.
Ulnar n. and a.
Median n. and a.
Sup. br. radial n.
Trans. carpal lig.

Deep palmar arch
Sup. palmar arch
Common volar digital n.

Gluteus maximus mus.
Gluteus medius mus.
Sup. gluteal n.
Piriformis mus.
Sacrotuberous lig.
Adductor magnus mus.
Iliotibial tract
Biceps femoris long head
Semitendinosus mus.
Biceps femoris short head
Common peroneal n.
Tibial n.
Lat. cutaneous sural n.
Plantaris mus.
Med. cutaneous sural n.
Gastrocnemius mus.

Vena cava
Aorta
Lumbar plexus T12-L4
Sacral plexus L4-S3
L5 vert.

Inf. gluteal n.
S4N
Coccygeal nn.
Sciatic n.
Pudendal n.
Post. femoral cutaneous n.
Tuberosity of ilium
Semimembranosus mus.
Popliteal a. and v.
Gracilis tendon
Small saphenous v.

Sympathetic n. trunk
Iliohypogastric n.
Ilioinguinal n.
Genitofemoral n.
Lat. femoral cutaneous n.
Accessory obturator n.
Obturator n.
Lumbosacral trunk
Branches for quadriceps femoris
Obturator n. ant. br.
Femoral a., v., n.
Adductor longus mus.
Saphenous n., femoral a. and v.
Adductor hiatus
Infrapatellar br.

Posterior View

Anterior View

leg, extension of the lower leg (femoral), and adduction and outward rotation of the leg (obturator).

The sacral plexus. The five pairs of sacral nerves form the posterior primary division, which gives medial and lateral branches to the multifidae muscles; the lateral branches also supply the skin over the medial part of the gluteus maximus. The anterior primary divisions form part of the lumbosacral plexus. The white rami (parasympathetic) and the gray rami (sympathetic) form part of the sacral nerves, the first passing from the second, third, and fourth sacral nerves to the pelvic and lower abdominal viscera through the hypogastric plexus, and the second joining each sacral nerve from the sympathetic trunk.

The sacral plexus lies against the piriformis muscle on the posterior wall of the pelvis. Several structures like the colon and hypogastric muscles lie in front of it. The sacral plexus is formed by the fourth and fifth lumbar nerves, and the first, second, and third sacral nerves. The upper four posterior divisions (L4–L5–S1–S2) are fused to form the common peroneal nerve; all five of the anterior divisions (L4–L5–S1–S2–S3) participate in the formation of the tibial nerves. The posterior division of S3 with some branches of the anterior divisions of S2 and S3 participate in the formation of the pudendal plexus. The sacral plexus (L5–S5) forms the origin of (1) the superior gluteal nerve (to the gluteus maximus, medius, and minimus; tensor fasciae latae; and piriformis muscles), serving abduction and inward rotation of the leg, flexion and extension of the leg at the hip, and outward rotation of the leg; (2) the inferior gluteal and sciatic nerves (obturator internus, gemellar, quadratus femoris, biceps femoris, semitendinosus, and semimembranosus muscles), serving outward rotation and flexion of the leg at the hip; (3) the peroneal nerve with two branches, the deep innervating the tibialis anterior, extensor digitorum longus, and extensor hallucis brevis muscles, which dorsiflex and supinate the foot and extend the toes, and the superficial innervating the peroneus muscle (pronation of the foot); (4) the tibial nerve (to the gastrocnemius, soleus, posterior tibial muscles, and flexors of the toes), responsible for the plantar flexion of the foot; (5) the pudendal nerve, innervating the perineal muscles and the sphincters, being responsible for the closure of sphincters of the pelvic organs, contraction of the pelvic floor, and participation in the sexual act.

The sensory innervation of the skin is either related to a proximal, dermatomic (root) or to a distal, cutaneous (peripheral nerve) distribution as illustrated in Plate 19. By charting the sensory deficit, the site of lesion or disease can be localized. It is of considerable importance that there is an overlap of three to five segments to any given dermatome. To denervate completely the dermatomic area on the skin, two segments above and two segments below the given area have to be denervated to produce complete anesthesia in a given segment.

Different grades of sensory disturbances from hypesthesia to complete anesthesia involving either the cutaneous radicular or the peripheral nerve fields may be present. Irritative phenomena, like spontaneous pains or dysesthesias, may be present, indicating overstimulation of sensory modalities along root distribution or in the territory of a peripheral nerve. These pains and dysesthesias, when they originate from an irritable focus in a posterior spinal root, are projected through the corresponding peripheral nerves. The brain will perceive, as source of the incoming pain, the area of the dermatome that is supplied by the affected spinal root. The anatomical regions to which pains are projected when a spinal root is involved are well defined. For example, irritation of the second lumbar root will result in the pain being projected to the anterior aspect of the thigh; the third lumbar root is projected into the middle anterior aspect of the thigh and the inner knee; the fourth lumbar root to the lateral aspect of the thigh, front and medial side of the leg and in the great toe; the fifth lumbar root to the lateral side of the leg, dorsal and lateral sole of the foot, and so on.

It is of interest that the sciatic nerve is the largest in the body. In the thigh, one sheet surrounds the two separate nerves, the common peroneal and the tibial nerves. The course of the sciatic nerve after leaving the pelvis to the greater sciatic foramen, usually below the piriformis muscle, is between the greater trochanter of the femur and the tuberosities of the ischia, along the posterior surface of the thigh, and then to the popliteal space, where it terminates by dividing into the tibial and common peroneal nerves.

The Central Nervous System

Melvin H. Epstein, M.D.
Donlin M. Long, M.D.

THE BRAIN

The brain can be divided into three major parts: the brain stem, the cerebellum, and the cerebrum. The brain stem can be further subdivided into medulla, pons, and midbrain. The medulla is that part of the brain which joins the brain to the spinal cord. The pons and midbrain are successively more rostral.

Gross Anatomy

The cerebrum is the newest part of the brain and that part which is responsible for highest mental function. The cerebrum is subdivided into lobes, four in all on each side. Grossly, the brain is exactly the same on both right and left, while functionally there are differences between the right side of the brain and the left. Most anterior are the frontal lobes, next come the parietal lobes, and the most posterior lobes are the occipital. The temporal lobe is tucked like the thumb of a mitten into the area just above the ear. Each of these lobes has special functions.

The outermost surface of the brain is composed of nerve cells and is called the *cortex*. The processes of these nerve cells passing upward and downward comprise the white matter, which is the greatest volume of the brain. Deep inside the brain, just above the brain stem, are several masses of nerve cells with very important functions. The most important of these is the thalamus, which is a way station for relay of messages to the cortex and has important functions in processing information as well. Another of these buried areas of gray matter is the hypothalamus, which has important connections in behavior and in hormone function. The third of these areas of nerve cells is called the *basal ganglia*. These cells are very important in coordination of motor movement.

The cerebrum sits on the brain stem, and the cerebellum, especially important in coordination of motor movement, is located in the angle between the brain stem and cerebrum. The brain stem has many important functions. Most of the cranial nerves come from the brain stem, and all of the fiber tracts passing up and down from peripheral nerves and spinal cord to the higher parts of the brain must traverse the brain stem. The brain stem is especially important in control of subconscious and reflex activities such as breathing, heart rate, and blood pressure.

The Cerebrospinal Fluid

If the brain is cut in cross section, it is seen to have four cavities within it. Inside the cerebrum there are large lateral ventricles that connect in the midline to the third ventricle. The third ventricle is connected by a very narrow passage called the *aqueduct* to the fourth ventricle, which lies between the brain stem and cerebellum. Within these ventricles a structure called the *choroid plexus* is located. The choroid plexus produces the cerebrospinal fluid, which is a clear, watery fluid that both supports the brain and provides its extracellular fluid. This fluid circulates through the ventricles, leaves the fourth ventricle, and descends in the spinal canal to circulate around the spinal cord and the spinal nerves, returning upward to pass over the entire surface of the brain to be absorbed into the veins.

Functional Anatomy of the Brain

The frontal lobes are important in two major areas. The anterior portion of the frontal lobe is called the *prefrontal cortex* and is especially important in highest mental function and in the determination of personality. The posterior part of the frontal lobe controls motor movement and is divided into a premotor and motor area. In the motor cortex are located the nerve cells that actually produce movement, and in the premotor area are several portions of the brain that modify movement. The frontal lobe is divided from the parietal lobe by the central sulcus. Immediately behind the motor cortex is the primary sensory cortex. This controls sensation such as touch, pressure, and localization of objects that touch the skin. Just behind this primary sensory area is a very large association area that controls such fine sensation as judgment of texture, weight, size, and shape.

The occipital lobe is concerned with vision. On the medial surface of the occipital lobe is located the calcarine cortex, which contains the cells that have to do with primary visual reception. The remainder of the occipital lobes are association areas that help in the recognition of size and shape and color.

The temporal lobe has numerous important functions. The auditory cortex is located on the superior internal portion of the temporal lobe and an area called the *hippocampus* forms the lobe's medial portion. This hippocampus and related structures are very important in behavior. The medial part of the temporal lobe is connected to the hypothalamus and then to the frontal lobes, with interconnections to many other parts of the brain.

On the left side of the brain in right-handed individuals is located the speech area. The hemisphere containing speech is called the *dominant hemisphere*. Motor speech is located at the base of the frontal lobe, in Broca's area. This is the part of the brain that controls the movement necessary for speech. On the lateral portion of the temporal lobe there is an important area that has to do with hearing speech, and in the base of the parietal lobe are association areas that have to do with understanding and carrying out the complex actions required for speech.

The portion of the brain most responsible for behavior is called the *limbic lobe*. The limbic lobe is not an anatomical lobe of the brain but a functional subdivision.

Blood Supply of the Brain

The brain gets its primary blood supply from the two internal carotid arteries and the two vertebral arteries. The vascular connections at the base of the brain form the circle of Willis, which is composed of a vascular loop consisting of the two anterior cerebral arteries and the anterior communicating artery in front and the posterior communicating artery and the posterior cerebral arteries behind. There are numerous variations and congenital abnormalities associated with the circle of Willis.

The internal carotid artery divides intracranially into two main branches. One is the anterior cerebral artery, which passes forward and immediately above the optic chiasm to enter the longitudinal fissure of the cerebrum. It furnishes blood to the major part of the medial aspect of the cerebral hemisphere and gives off several vital perforating branches at the base of the brain that supply blood to the head of the caudate, the anterior part of the lentiform nucleus, the internal capsule, the anterior columns of the fornix, and the anterior commissures. The loss of these important perforators leads to deep coma.

The middle cerebral artery is the larger of the two terminal branches of the internal carotid artery and passes laterally through the Sylvian fissure to the surface of the insula, where it divides into numerous parietal and temporal cortical branches. During its course through the Sylvian fissure it gives off important perforating arteries called *medial* and *lateral striate arteries,* which pass upward through the putamen of the lentiform nucleus, and it also supplies blood to the globus pallidus and the internal capsule. These arteries that frequently rupture in cases of spontaneous cerebral hemorrhage are known as the *arteries of Charcot.*

The vertebral arteries enter the intracranial cavity and traverse the base of the medulla, giving off two posteroinferior cerebellar arteries, which supply blood to the brain stem and the posteroinferior surface of the cerebellum. The vertebral arteries then join to become the basilar artery. The important perforating branches from the basilar artery to the remainder of the brain stem are vital to many life functions. The anteroinferior cerebellar artery arises from the basilar artery at the ponto-medullary junction and gives blood to the anteroinferior surfaces of the cerebellum. There is frequently an important loop that passes into the internal auditory canal from the anteroinferior cerebellar artery and returns to the brain stem to supply blood to the pons. Close to the basilar summit arises the superior cerebellar artery, which has perforating branches to the brain stem and to the superior surface of the cerebellum.

The posterior cerebral arteries are the terminal branches of the basilar system. They also have extremely important perforating central arteries, which supply blood to the cerebral peduncle, the posterior perforated substance, the posterior part of the thalamus, and the mammillary bodies during their course around the brain stem. The posterior choroidal branches pass through the upper part of the choroid fissure, then to the posterior part of the tela choroidea of the third ventricle, and then to the choroid plexus. The posterior cerebral supplies blood to the uncus, hippocampal gyrus, medial temporal lobe, occipital pole, and to a small portion of the posterior parietal lobe.

Plate 21.
The Five Senses of Consciousness

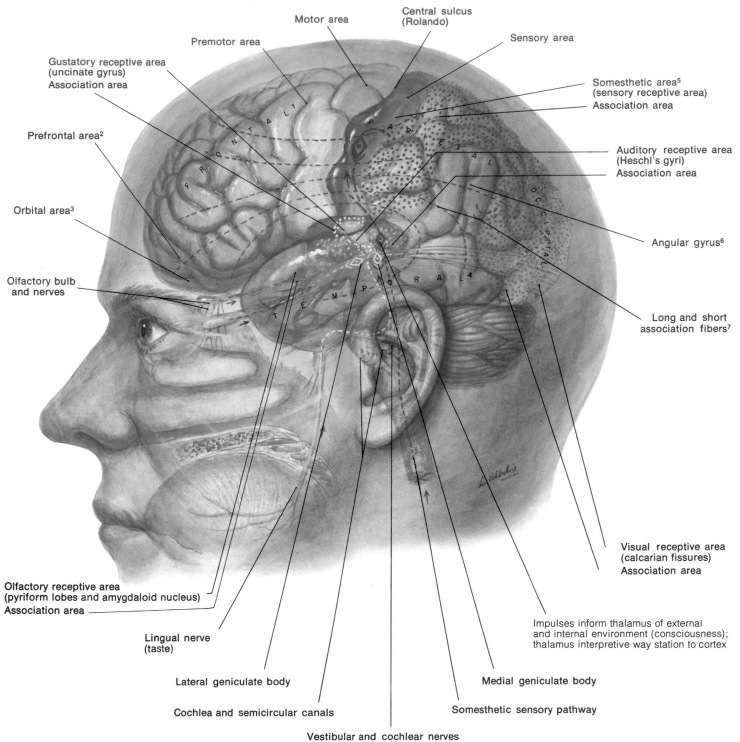

Motor area

Central sulcus (Rolando)

Premotor area

Sensory area

Gustatory receptive area (uncinate gyrus)
Association area

Somesthetic area[5] (sensory receptive area)
Association area

Prefrontal area[2]

Auditory receptive area (Heschl's gyri)
Association area

Orbital area[3]

Angular gyrus[6]

Olfactory bulb and nerves

Long and short association fibers[7]

Visual receptive area (calcarian fissures)
Association area

Olfactory receptive area (pyriform lobes and amygdaloid nucleus)
Association area

Impulses inform thalamus of external and internal environment (consciousness); thalamus interpretive way station to cortex

Lingual nerve (taste)

Lateral geniculate body

Medial geniculate body

Cochlea and semicircular canals

Somesthetic sensory pathway

Vestibular and cochlear nerves

[1] Frontal lobe
Controls personality stability, ambitions, responsibilities, and properties of behavior

[2] Prefrontal area
Relatively high association evaluation and control of emotion, judgment, and conduct, and center for complex motor capabilities

[3] Orbital regions
General areas of autonomic control presiding over hypothalamus to control basic rhythms of life

[4] Temporal lobe
Basic intellectual, emotional and sexual activities

[5] Somesthetic area
Evaluation of muscular activity and interpretation of touch and other physical properties

[6] Angular gyrus
Visual speech center (symbolic communication); ability to recognize the written word

[7] Long and short association fibers
link together various primary association (memory) sensation areas into more complex memories.

Plate 22.
Vascular Supply of the Brain

Sup. sagittal sinus

Middle cerebral v.

Ant. communicating a.

Ant. cerebral a.

Middle cerebral a.

Frontopolar a.

Post. communicating a.

Cavernous sinus

Ophthalmic a.

Int. carotid a.

Basilar a.

Vertebral a.

Ext. carotid a.

Int. jugular v.

Sup. and inf. orbital vv.

Inf. sagittal sinus

Sup. cerebellar a.

Sup. anastomotic v. (Trolard's)

Sup. cerebral v.

Great cerebral v.

Straight sinus

Transverse sinus

Occipital sinus

Inf. anastomotic v. of Labbé

Emissary v.

Sigmoid sinus

Post. inf. cerebellar a.

Vertebral a. thru foramina of 2nd & 3rd vert.

Post. cerebral a.

Inf. auditory a.

Ant. int. cerebellar a.

Carotid sinus

Sup. sagittal sinus

Lat. ventricle

Foramen of Monro

III ventricle

Cist. Sylvii

Cist. suprasellar

Cist. interpeduncularis

Inf. horn lat. vent.

Temporal lobe

Cist. pontis

Foramen of Luschka

Filum terminale

Choroid plexus

Arachnoid granulations

Aqueduct of Sylvius

Post. horn lat. vent.

Cist. great cerebral v.

Cist. quadrigemina

Cerebellum

IV ventricle

Cist. magna

Foramen of Magendie

Central canal of cord

Subarachnoid space

CIRCULATION OF CEREBROSPINAL FLUID

CEREBRAL CISTERNAE

Cist. callosi

III ventricle

Lat. ventricle

Cist. quadrigemina

Cist. great cerebral v.

Aqueduct of Sylvius

IV ventricle

Cist. lamina terminalis

Cist. Sylvii

Cist. chiasmatica

Cist. suprasellar

Cist. ambiens

Cist. interpeduncularis

Cist. pontis

Cist. medullaris

Cist. magna

The Cranial Nerves

The olfactory nerve, or first cranial nerve, is the pathway taken by olfactory impulses from the nasal mucosa to the brain. The olfactory tract connects the olfactory bulb with the olfactory tubercle, where it divides into a medial and lateral olfactory tract. The optic nerve, or second cranial nerve, lies just posterior and inferior to the medial olfactory tract. It carries information from the eye for vision and ocular reflexes. The third cranial nerve, or oculomotor nerve, arises at the ventral aspect of the mesencephalon and transverses through the cavernous sinus to the orbit. It supplies all the intrinsic ocular muscles and all extrinsic ocular muscles except for the lateral rectus and superior oblique. The parasympathetic fibers from this nerve innervate the ciliary muscle of the lens and the sphincter muscle of the pupil. The fourth, or trochlear, nerve supplies only the superior oblique muscle of the eye, and it arises just below the inferior quadrigeminal bodies of the brain stem. It emerges from the posterior aspect of the brain stem and passes around the lateral side of the cerebral peduncle into the margin of the tentorium and into the cavernous sinus, where it goes to the orbit. The fifth cranial nerve, or trigeminal nerve, is the largest cranial nerve, and it carries fibers that give sensation to the face and motor fibers to the muscles of mastication. It exits from the brain stem through the anterolateral surface of the pons.

The sixth, or abducent, nerve supplies the lateral rectus muscle of the eyeball and issues from the brain at the inferior border of the pons, just above the pyramid of the medulla. The seventh, or facial, nerve consists of two parts: the motor root, which supplies the superficial muscles of the scalp, face, and neck; and a smaller sensory root, which contains the afferent taste fibers for the anterior two thirds of the tongue and the afferent parasympathetic fibers for supply of the lacrimal and salivary glands. The facial nerve arises from the lateral aspect of the pontomedullary junction. The auditory nerve, or eighth nerve, is entirely sensory and consists of vestibular and cochlear divisions. The glossopharyngeal, or ninth, nerve is a mixed nerve consisting of an afferent part, which supplies the pharynx and tongue and the carotid sinus and body, and the efferent part, which supplies the stylopharyngeus muscle. It arises from the medulla by five or six fine rootlets which are attached to the side of the medulla oblongata, close to the facial nerve.

The vagus, or tenth, nerve is also a mixed nerve, which contains a large number of parasympathetic fibers and passes through the neck and thorax into the abdomen. It supplies afferent fibers chiefly to the pharynx, esophagus, stomach, larynx, trachea, and lungs. It is attached by numerous rootlets to the side of the medulla, in series with the glossopharyngeal nerve above and the accessory nerve below. The rootlets unite to form a single tract which exits from the cranial cavity through the jugular foramen. The accessory nerve, or eleventh cranial nerve, consists of bulbar and spinal portions. It arises in series with the vagus and glossopharyngeal nerve and controls motor function of the sternomastoid and the trapezius muscles. The twelfth, or hypoglossal, nerve is a predominantly efferent nerve that supplies all the muscles of the tongue, both intrinsic and extrinsic, except the palatoglossus muscle. It arises from numerous rootlets from the anterior portion of the medulla oblongata. The rootlets arrange themselves in double bundles and unite in the anterior condylar canal, where they emerge from the cranial cavity.

Circulation of Cerebral Spinal Fluid

Most of the cerebral spinal fluid is formed within the lateral ventricles of the brain by the choroid plexus. Cerebral spinal fluid is a clear, colorless liquid of low specific gravity that in health has between two and three lymphocytes per cubic millimeter. Its total volume is between 100 and 140 ml in adults, and the normal pressure varies from between 70 and 200 mm of water with the patient on his side. Total protein in the adult varies from 20 to 45 mg percent, with glucose varying from 50 to 75 mg percent. Chlorides are between 120 and 230 m eq/lit.

From the lateral ventricles, fluid traverses the interventricular foramina into the third ventricle. Here, presumably, the choroid plexus of the third ventricle contributes fluid, which then passes through the aqueduct of Sylvius into the fourth ventricle, where further additions are made by the choroid plexus in the roof of the fourth ventricle. The fluid then escapes into the subarachnoid space through a median aperture called the *foramen of Magendie* and lateral apertures called *foramina of Luschka*. Some fluid passes downward into the spinal subarachnoid space, but the major portion rises through the tentorial notch and finds its way slowly over the surface of the hemispheres to be absorbed mainly through the arachnoid villi and granulations into the venous system. There appear to be other mechanisms of CSF absorption, mainly through the perineural lymphatics, and, in addition, in abnormal pressure states it appears possible for CSF to be absorbed through the ependyma. Each blood vessel, as it enters the brain tissue, incorporates a prolongation of the subarachnoid space by which cerebrospinal fluid can come in contact with the neurons themselves. Any obstruction to the ventricular system, either by blockage of the foramen of Monro, the aqueduct of Sylvius, or of the foramina of Magendie and Luschka, will create a non-communicating type

Plate 23.
Base of the Brain and of the Skull

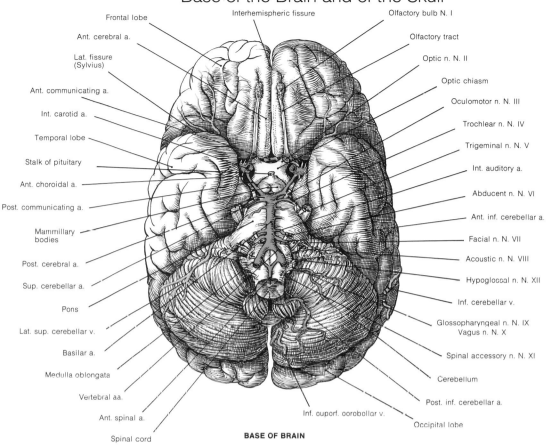

Frontal lobe
Ant. cerebral a.
Lat. fissure (Sylvius)
Ant. communicating a.
Int. carotid a.
Temporal lobe
Stalk of pituitary
Ant. choroidal a.
Post. communicating a.
Mammillary bodies
Post. cerebral a.
Sup. cerebellar a.
Pons
Lat. sup. cerebellar v.
Basilar a.
Medulla oblongata
Vertebral aa.
Ant. spinal a.
Spinal cord

Interhemispheric fissure

Olfactory bulb N. I
Olfactory tract
Optic n. N. II
Optic chiasm
Oculomotor n. N. III
Trochlear n. N. IV
Trigeminal n. N. V
Int. auditory a.
Abducent n. N. VI
Ant. inf. cerebellar a.
Facial n. N. VII
Acoustic n. N. VIII
Hypoglossal n. N. XII
Inf. cerebellar v.
Glossopharyngeal n. N. IX
Vagus n. N. X
Spinal accessory n. N. XI
Cerebellum
Post. inf. cerebellar a.
Inf. superf. cerebellar v.
Occipital lobe

BASE OF BRAIN

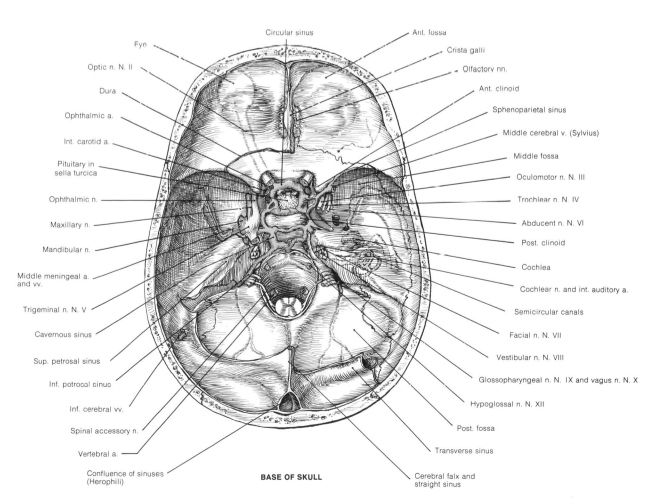

Eye
Optic n. N. II
Dura
Ophthalmic a.
Int. carotid a.
Pituitary in sella turcica
Ophthalmic n.
Maxillary n.
Mandibular n.
Middle meningeal a. and vv.
Trigeminal n. N. V
Cavernous sinus
Sup. petrosal sinus
Inf. petrosal sinus
Inf. cerebral vv.
Spinal accessory n.
Vertebral a.
Confluence of sinuses (Herophili)

Circular sinus
Ant. fossa
Crista galli
Olfactory nn.
Ant. clinoid
Sphenoparietal sinus
Middle cerebral v. (Sylvius)
Middle fossa
Oculomotor n. N. III
Trochlear n. N. IV
Abducent n. N. VI
Post. clinoid
Cochlea
Cochlear n. and int. auditory a.
Semicircular canals
Facial n. N. VII
Vestibular n. N. VIII
Glossopharyngeal n. N. IX and vagus n. N. X
Hypoglossal n. N. XII
Post. fossa
Transverse sinus
Cerebral falx and straight sinus

BASE OF SKULL

of hydrocephalus in which the ventricular system will dilate. The pressure within the ventricular system in hydrocephalus can increase in an acute and fatal manner. If absorption is interfered with, there develops a hydrocephalus that is classified as communicating.

THE SPINAL CORD

The spinal cord is a continuation of the lower part of the brain stem, which descends in the bony vertebral column giving off thirty-one pairs of nerves. The spinal cord ends between the first and second lumbar vertebral bodies as the conus medullaris. Below this level the nerve roots are called the *cauda equina.*

The spinal cord is divided into anterior and posterior halves. This division is recognized by the dentate ligaments, which attach the lateral sides of the spinal cord to the surrounding dura. The posterior half of the spinal cord is further divided by the posterior median longitudinal fissure. The posterior spinal roots enter the spinal cord at approximately the midpoint of this posterior quadrant. The anterior half of the spinal cord is also divided by the anterior longitudinal fissure, which runs down the midline. In this fissure is located the anterior spinal artery, which is the major blood supply to the spinal cord. The anterior spinal roots arise from the anterior quadrant and pass laterally to join the posterior spinal roots at the dura mater, to continue outward as peripheral nerves. Each of these small roots is made up of several rootlets, which join together to form the roots. There are eight cervical nerves on each side, twelve thoracic, five lumbar, and five sacral. The small coccygeal that makes the thirty-first pair is inconstant. A long fibrous structure called the *filum terminale* attaches the conus medullaris to the sacrum. In the cervical region and at the lower end of the spinal cord, the spinal cord swells as the cervical and lumbar enlargements. These are the areas where the large nerves that make up the brachial plexus and the lumbosacral plexus arise. These plexuses provide the supply of sensation and movement to the arms and legs.

The blood supply of the spinal cord comes primarily from the anterior spinal artery, which arises from the vertebral artery and then descends in the anterior median sulcus. At many levels in the spinal cord, small blood vessels enter with the nerve roots and anastomose with the anterior spinal artery.

Functional Anatomy of the Spinal Cord

The posterior medial portions of the spinal cord are called the *posterior columns.* These transmit such sensations as position, joint sense, and pressure.

Lateral to the posterior columns, but still behind the dentate ligament, are located the corticospinal tracts. These are the motor tracts that control movement. The outer portion of the spinal cord is white matter, and the nerve cells or gray matter are located internally, in structures called *horns.* In front of the dentate ligament in the anterior quadrants are located the anterior horns. The large nerve cells of the anterior horns are the final common path for all motor activity and supply the impulses that cause movement in all muscles of the body except those supplied by the cranial nerves. The nerve cells that have to do with sensation are in the posterior portion of the spinal cord and are called the *posterior horns.*

The spinal cord is surrounded by a tough fibrous structure called the *dura mater.* This covers the spinal cord and all of the spinal nerves. The spinal nerves exit from the spinal cord, pierce the dura, and descend to reach the nearest neural foramen. The foramen is the opening between the vertebral bodies through which the nerves exit. In this foramen is located a small structure called the *dorsal root ganglion,* in which the cells that supply sensation to the body are located. As soon as the nerve leaves the bony protection of the neural foramen, it is termed a *peripheral nerve.* The spinal nerves are numbered according to the vertebral body with which they are associated. In the cervical region, all of the nerves leave above the vertebral body of the same number except the eighth cervical nerve, which exits below the body of the seventh vertebra. Below that level all of the nerves exit below the vertebral body of the same number.

It is possible to locate the area of the spinal cord by the relations of the spinal segments with the vertebra. Between the level of the second cervical and the tenth thoracic spinous processes, adding two to the number of the spinous process felt will give the underlying spinal cord segment. The eleventh and twelfth spinous processes overlie the five lumbar segments and the first lumbar spinous process overlies the five sacral segments.

Plate 24.
Cerebrospinal Axis and Cervical Cord

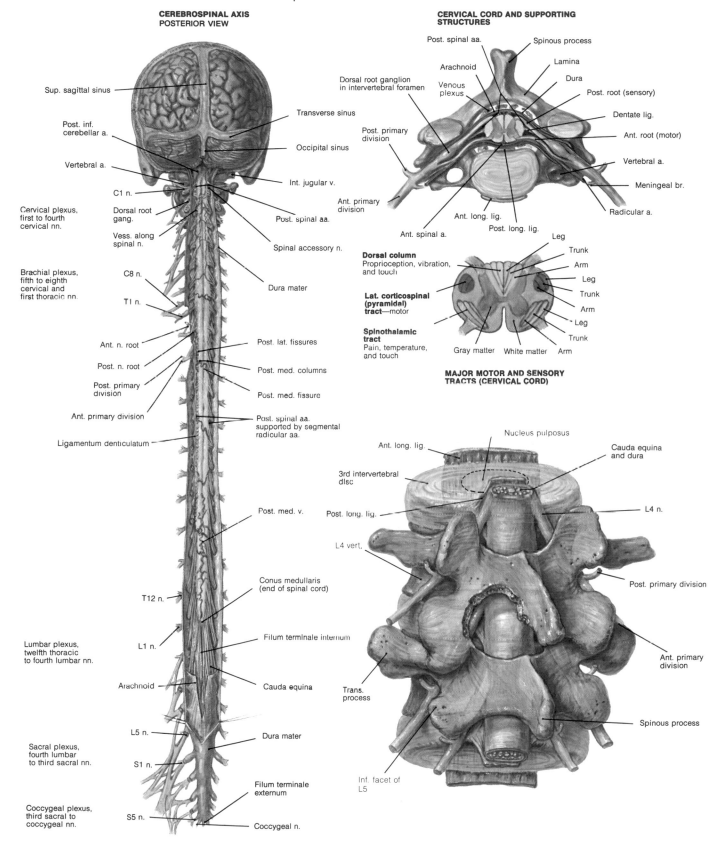

CEREBROSPINAL AXIS POSTERIOR VIEW

- Sup. sagittal sinus
- Post. inf. cerebellar a.
- Vertebral a.
- C1 n.
- Cervical plexus, first to fourth cervical nn.
- Dorsal root gang.
- Vess. along spinal n.
- Brachial plexus, fifth to eighth cervical and first thoracic nn.
- C8 n.
- TI n.
- Ant. n. root
- Post. n. root
- Post. primary division
- Ant. primary division
- Ligamentum denticulatum
- T12 n.
- Lumbar plexus, twelfth thoracic to fourth lumbar nn.
- L1 n.
- Arachnoid
- L5 n.
- Sacral plexus, fourth lumbar to third sacral nn.
- S1 n.
- Coccygeal plexus, third sacral to coccygeal nn.
- S5 n.

- Transverse sinus
- Occipital sinus
- Int. jugular v.
- Post. spinal aa.
- Spinal accessory n.
- Dura mater
- Post. lat. fissures
- Post. med. columns
- Post. med. fissure
- Post. spinal aa. supported by segmental radicular aa.
- Post. med. v.
- Conus medullaris (end of spinal cord)
- Filum terminale internum
- Cauda equina
- Dura mater
- Filum terminale externum
- Coccygeal n.

CERVICAL CORD AND SUPPORTING STRUCTURES

- Post. spinal aa.
- Arachnoid
- Venous plexus
- Dorsal root ganglion in intervertebral foramen
- Post. primary division
- Ant. primary division
- Ant. long. lig.
- Ant. spinal a.
- Spinous process
- Lamina
- Dura
- Post. root (sensory)
- Dentate lig.
- Ant. root (motor)
- Vertebral a.
- Meningeal br.
- Radicular a.
- Ant. long. lig.
- Post. long. lig.

Dorsal column
Proprioception, vibration, and touch

Lat. corticospinal (pyramidal) tract—motor

Spinothalamic tract
Pain, temperature, and touch

- Leg
- Trunk
- Arm
- Leg
- Trunk
- Arm
- Leg
- Trunk
- Arm
- Gray matter
- White matter

MAJOR MOTOR AND SENSORY TRACTS (CERVICAL CORD)

- Nucleus pulposus
- Ant. long. lig.
- 3rd intervertebral disc
- L4 vert.
- Trans. process
- Inf. facet of L5
- Cauda equina and dura
- L4 n.
- Post. primary division
- Ant. primary division
- Spinous process

The Lymphatic System

James P. Isaacs, M.D.

The lymphatic system originates embryonically from transformed venous endothelium as a series of paired and unpaired sacs. The jugular and sciatic lymphatic sacs are paired, arising respectively from jugular and iliac veins; the retroperitoneal sac, unpaired, arises from the inferior vena cava and mesonephric veins. The unpaired cisterna chyli, which originates from the Wolffian ducts, becomes the drainage center for retroperitoneal and sciatic lymphatic sacs, jejunal and ileal fatty lymphatics or lacteals, and bilateral descending intercostal lymphatic trunks. The cisterna chyli occupies a strategic retroperitoneal position in the right upper lumbar paravertebral gutter. The thoracic duct empties the cisterna chyli, passing through the diaphragm into the right chest, crossing into the left chest at the fifth thoracic vertebra, and extending to the lower left neck. Here it drains into the junction of the left subclavian and internal jugular veins. Near this venous junction on the left or right side of the neck, three lymphatic trunks (subclavian, inferior jugular, and bronchomediastinal) join the thoracic duct or right lymphatic duct respectively.

Musculature is present in the walls of lymphatic trunks and ducts in increasing amounts as these vessels get larger. Contraction of this intrinsic muscle in the presence of one-way valves exerts a pumping action on the lymph. Contraction of surrounding muscle masses also assists in lymph pumping. Lymph flow rate from the thoracic duct terminus is 50 to 100 cc per hour at a rest pressure near zero. The thoracic duct pressure and flow rise sensitively with exercise, increased body temperature, and alimentation.

The lymphatic system is also a defense system with limited capacity. When pathologically overwhelmed, it is a route for spread of bacterial infections, parasitic infestations, tumor metastases, foreign body contaminations, inflammatory degenerations, and chemical absorptions. The lymphatics can be obstructed by accumulation of particulate materials, by lymphangitis, and by lymph clotting, thrombosis, and embolization. The lymphatic valves are injured in the same manner that venous valves are injured by phlebitis and venous thrombosis. Traumatic division of larger lymphatic vessels also occurs. The various obstructions and divisions create troublesome or sometimes fatal syndromes, which include chyle thorax, chyle peritoneum, and lymphedema of extremities, genitourinary organs, and so forth.

The lymphatic system has other forms of pathology: neoplasia (Hodgkin's disease, lymphomas, lymphosarcoma, cystic hygroma, etc.) and metaplasia and hyperplasia (pyogenic, granulomatous, and other infections). Some lymphatic vessels may be congenitally absent (congenital lymphedema).

The lymphatic system is an active component of the circulatory system that drains peripheral tissues in parallel with venous return.

Virtually all structures in the body possess a fine reticulum of blind-ended lymphatic channels which are lined by endothelial cells. These cells pass many different chemical and biological substances from tissues in the formation of lymph.

Lymph is an isotonic, relatively fat-rich, protein-poor fluid that is carried from its reticular origin through afferent tubular lymphatics to lymph nodes.

Each lymph node has an arterial blood supply and venous drainage, with lymphoid germinal centers that add lymphoid cells to circulating lymph and blood. Sinuses of each lymph node collect into an efferent tubule, which joins with other tubules to form larger lymphatic trunks. The trunks empty into two main lymphatic ducts, the thoracic duct and the right lymphatic duct.

Plate 25.
Lymphatics: Head, Neck, and Chest

Frontal a.

Zygomaticoörbital a.

Sup. temporal vess.

Trans. facial

Occipital a.

Ant. auricular and intraglandular parotid nodes

Occipital nodes

Parotid gland

Post. auricular nodes

Ext. maxillary a.

Superficial nodes

Submandibular nodes

Ant. facial v.

Submandibular gland

Ext. jugular v.

Submental nodes

Sup. deep lat. nodes

Sup. deep nodes (medial)

Superficial ant. nodes

Spinal accessory chain

Omohyoid mus.

Sternomastoid mus.

Sup. deep lat. nodes

Supraclavicular nodes

Int. jugular v.

To r. jugular lymphatic trunk

Thyroid gland

Post. deep temporal a.

Ant. deep temporal a.

Med. retropharyngeal nodes

Infraorbital a.

Middle meningeal a.

Int. maxillary a.

Lat. retropharyngeal nodes

Ext. maxillary a.

Asc. pharyngeal a.

Lingual a.

Ext. carotid a.

Sup. thyroid a.

Thyroid cart.

Common carotid a.

Pretracheal nodes

Subclavicular nodes

Deltoid pectoral

Axillary vess.

Pectoralis minor mus

Inf. retropharyngeal nodes

Interpectoral nodes of Rotter

Int. mammary nodes

Innominate v.

Recurrent laryngeal nn. and paratracheal nodes

Lat. thoracic vess.

Cephalic v.

Sup. vena cava

Lung

Axillary v. nodes

Azygos v.

Pectoralis major mus.

Tracheo-bronchial nodes

Sternal nodes

Scapular nodes and vess.

Phrenic n.

Central nodes

Aorta

Latissimus dorsi mus.

Pulm. a.

Mammary gland

Ext. mammary nodes

Ant. diaph. nodes

Middle diaph. nodes

Plate 26.
Lymphatics: Esophagus and Stomach; Colon, Rectum, and Anus

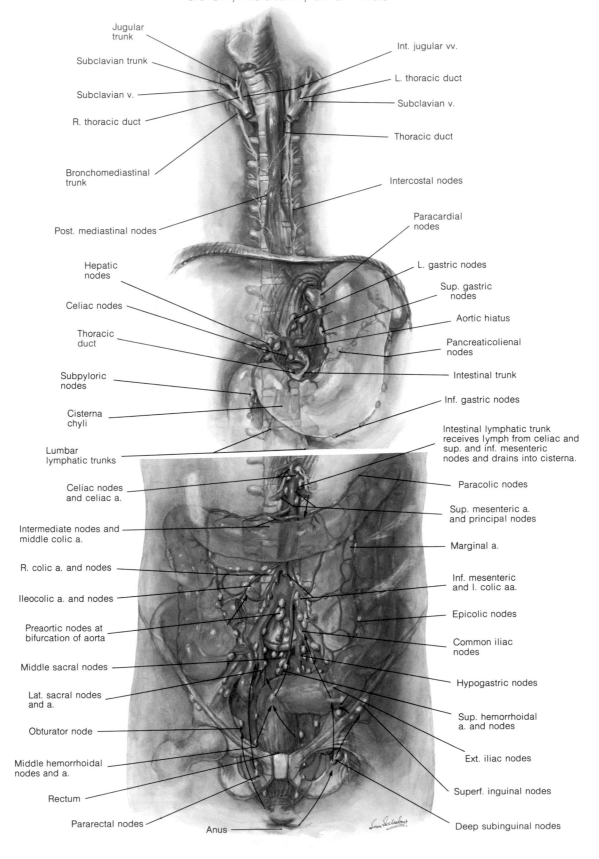

Jugular trunk

Subclavian trunk

Subclavian v.

R. thoracic duct

Bronchomediastinal trunk

Post. mediastinal nodes

Hepatic nodes

Celiac nodes

Thoracic duct

Subpyloric nodes

Cisterna chyli

Lumbar lymphatic trunks

Celiac nodes and celiac a.

Intermediate nodes and middle colic a.

R. colic a. and nodes

Ileocolic a. and nodes

Preaortic nodes at bifurcation of aorta

Middle sacral nodes

Lat. sacral nodes and a.

Obturator node

Middle hemorrhoidal nodes and a.

Rectum

Pararectal nodes

Anus

Int. jugular vv.

L. thoracic duct

Subclavian v.

Thoracic duct

Intercostal nodes

Paracardial nodes

L. gastric nodes

Sup. gastric nodes

Aortic hiatus

Pancreaticolienal nodes

Intestinal trunk

Inf. gastric nodes

Intestinal lymphatic trunk receives lymph from celiac and sup. and inf. mesenteric nodes and drains into cisterna.

Paracolic nodes

Sup. mesenteric a. and principal nodes

Marginal a.

Inf. mesenteric and l. colic aa.

Epicolic nodes

Common iliac nodes

Hypogastric nodes

Sup. hemorrhoidal a. and nodes

Ext. iliac nodes

Superf. inguinal nodes

Deep subinguinal nodes

Plate 27.
Lymphatics: Genitourinary System;
Liver and Bile Ducts

Medial aortic nodes

Spermatic vein

Sacral nodes

Vas deferens and seminal vesicle

Superficial inguinal nodes

Lymph node of Cloquet

Bladder

Deep subinguinal nodes

Prostate

Membranous urethra

Epididymis and testis

Glans penis

Adrenal

Kidney

Celiac and superior mesenteric nodes (preaortic)

Lateral aortic nodes

Inferior mesenteric nodes (preaortic)

Common iliac nodes

Ureter

Hypogastric nodes

External iliac nodes

Superficial inguinal nodes

Uterine and vaginal nodes

Uterine vessels

Ureter

Vaginal orifice

Inferior vena cava nodes

Superficial lymphatic vessels

Celiac nodes

Stomach

Liver

Spleen

Cystic nodes

Superior gastric nodes

Pancreaticolienal nodes

Hepatic nodes

Subpyloric nodes

Pancreas

Duodenum

The Eye and the Mechanism of Vision

Charles E. Iliff, M.D.

THE LIDS, EXTRAOCULAR
MUSCLES, AND LACRIMAL APPARATUS

The eye is surrounded by the bones of the skull on all sides except the front, where it is protected by the lids. The lids contain a platelike fibrous tissue—the tarsus—which gives inner support and added substance to this partially muscular curtain.

The lids are fastened nasally and laterally to the bony orbital wall by fibrous ligaments, so that when the orbicularis muscle contracts, the lid fissure is closed. This motion is voluntary in the wink and is reflex in the blink; these mechanisms are important in helping protect the globe from injury and for the lubrication of the cornea by spreading of tears, mucus, and other secretions from the glands of the conjunctiva. The lids are opened by the levator palpebrae muscle, which is the primary retractor of the upper lid, and by the secondary elevators of the lid: Müller's muscle, the superior rectus, and the frontalis muscle.

The eye rides in its bony socket on a cushion of fat through which run tendons, muscles, nerves, and blood vessels. The fat gently supports the globe, and the ligaments limit its motion.

Of the six extraocular muscles, the four recti have an origin around the optic foramen and insert on the sclera of the anterior portion of the globe. There are two oblique muscles. The superior oblique has its origin (with the four rectus muscles) at the annulus of Zinn, passes forward to the trochlea (pulley) on the anterior superonasal wall of the orbit, and from here passes beneath the superior rectus muscle and inserts into the sclera, temporal to and above the posterior pole of the globe. The inferior oblique muscle originates from the anterior orbital wall near the lacrimal fossa and passes backward to insert on the globe below the horizontal meridian and slightly temporal to the posterior pole. These six muscles working together give each globe its full range of motion, which permits the two eyes to work together and allows the visual axes to rotate as far as the limits provided by the orbital rims.

The lacrimal gland in the superotemporal quadrant of the orbit secretes tears (lacrimae), which lubricate the conjunctiva and cornea. The tears pass from the lacrimal ducts in the upper temporal conjunctiva and then across the globe to exit through the lacrimal puncta, the single small openings on the nasal edge of the upper and lower lid. The tears are normally kept from running over the lid margins by the fatty secretion from the Meibomian glands and glands of Moll, and are somewhat reduced in amount by evaporation as they pass to the lid puncta. Here they are funneled along the upper and lower lacrimal ducts into the lacrimal sacs, and from there through a bony canal to the mucous membrane of the nose, where they are evaporated by the air passing over the turbinates during respiration.

VASCULAR SUPPLY,
LYMPHATICS, AND MAJOR NERVES

The ophthalmic artery, a branch of the internal carotid artery, supplies most of the orbital structures, including the eye and its internal structures. There are a few branches of the internal maxillary artery that supply the inferior rectus and oblique muscles, the lacrimal sac and gland, and lower lid. The venous system mainly drains backward into the cavernous sinus, but there are also many anastomoses with the facial veins and veins of the nasal cavity.

The lids have lymphatic drainage channels, but

there are no lymphatics in the globe, and they are not normally found in the orbit. However, lymphangiomatous tumors do occur in the orbit, supposedly beginning in the lids and extending backward.

The nerves of the eye and orbit include the second cranial nerve—the optic nerve—which is actually an extension of the brain. The third cranial nerve—the oculomotor nerve—supplies the motor impulses for the levator muscles of the lid; the superior, medial, and inferior recti; and the inferior oblique muscles of the globe. The third nerve also sends off a motor root to the ciliary ganglion, which furnishes the autonomic innervation to the muscles within the globe, including the constrictor muscle of the iris.

The fourth and sixth cranial nerves are also motor nerves, and they supply the superior oblique and external rectus muscles respectively.

The fifth cranial nerve—the trigeminal—provides the sensory mechanism for the orbital structures, and in addition it supplies the surrounding area of the face and sinuses.

The seventh cranial nerve innervates the orbicularis muscles of the lids. The autonomic system controls the sphincter and dilator muscles of the pupil, the ciliary body, the operation of the lacrimal gland, and the smooth muscles of the lids and orbit.

ANATOMY OF THE EYE (THE GLOBE)

The globe itself measures about 24 mm in diameter. The anterior portion of the globe consists of the cornea, the curved transparent segment that is about 11 mm in diameter. The cornea is composed of avascular parallel layers of fibrous tissue, covered on the outside with epithelial cells and on the inside with endothelial cells. The posterior portion of the globe is the opaque sclera, which consists of a tough fibrous coat made up of connective tissue, elastic fibers, and blood vessels.

Behind the cornea is the anterior chamber, which is filled with a clear fluid, the aqueous humor. The posterior boundary of the anterior chamber consists of the crystalline lens and the iris. The lens is clear, and its shape is changed by the action of the ciliary muscle and by lens elasticity to enable the eye to focus on distant and near objects. The opening in the iris, the pupil, controls the amount of light entering the eye by the action of the constricting and dilating muscles of the iris. The lens is supported in the eye by fine fibers—the zonular fibers—which suspend the lens from the ciliary body. (These fibers, encircling the lens equator, are collectively called the zonules.) The ciliary body, in addition to being the base for the zonular fibers, secretes (or excretes) the aqueous fluid, which passes forward through the pupillary space into the anterior chamber and then exits through the trabecular meshwork and Schlemm's canal, which are located in the angle of the anterior chamber. The angle is formed by the attachment of the peripheral portion of the iris to the supporting sclera.

Just beneath the sclera, and lining the posterior portion of the globe, is the choroid, which carries the main vascular supply to the outer layers of the retina. The retina, which is a highly differentiated structure, with its receptor elements—the rods and cones—connects with the brain along the visual pathway of the optic nerve.The retina is a complex structure composed of an outer layer of pigment epithelium and an inner sensory epithelium. The sensory retina includes the rods and cones—the visual cells—which are supported by a connective tissue framework that carries ganglion cells, connecting cells, and nerve fibers; these fibers join to form the optic nerve, which carries the visual images to the brain. When the retina is observed with an ophthalmoscope, the optic nerve head (the optic disc) is seen as an oval structure with a pinkish hue, but of much lighter color than the surrounding retina. The ophthalmic artery and vein emerge from the nerve head to course over the retina and supply its superficial layers. The macula—a small central area containing a pit (the fovea), located near the posterior pole of the globe—is an area of the retina in which cones predominate and the rods are few; this is the area of most acute vision.

Within the cavity of the globe is the vitreous, which is a transparent, semigelatinous substance that provides an inner supporting structure central to the retina, choroid, ciliary body, and lens.

The optic nerve from each eye runs backward in the orbit and through the optic canal and then joins with the other optic nerve at the optic chiasm, where the temporal half of the fibers (from the lateral portion of retina) pass backward to the lateral geniculate body and from there to the visual cortex. The fibers from the nasal retina of each eye pass back to the optic chiasm and cross over (decussate) to the opposite optic tract (in an X-like manner) to join with the temporal fibers from the other eye, and with these fibers pass backward to the geniculate body and then to the visual cortex.

Plate 28.
The Eye and the Orbit

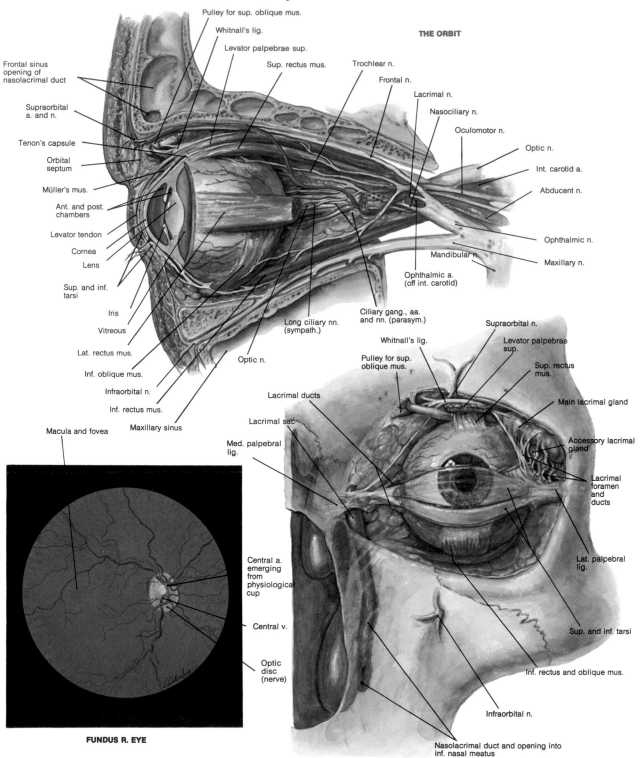

Pulley for sup. oblique mus.

Whitnall's lig.

Levator palpebrae sup.

Sup. rectus mus.

THE ORBIT

Trochlear n.

Frontal n.

Lacrimal n.

Nasociliary n.

Oculomotor n.

Optic n.

Int. carotid a.

Abducent n.

Ophthalmic n.

Mandibular n.

Maxillary n.

Ophthalmic a. (off int. carotid)

Frontal sinus opening of nasolacrimal duct

Supraorbital a. and n.

Tenon's capsule

Orbital septum

Müller's mus.

Ant. and post. chambers

Levator tendon

Cornea

Lens

Sup. and inf. tarsi

Iris

Vitreous

Lat. rectus mus.

Inf. oblique mus.

Infraorbital n.

Inf. rectus mus.

Optic n.

Long ciliary nn. (sympath.)

Ciliary gang., aa. and nn. (parasym.)

Maxillary sinus

Macula and fovea

Central a. emerging from physiological cup

Central v.

Optic disc (nerve)

FUNDUS R. EYE

Whitnall's lig.

Pulley for sup. oblique mus.

Lacrimal ducts

Lacrimal sac

Med. palpebral lig.

Supraorbital n.

Levator palpebrae sup.

Sup. rectus mus.

Main lacrimal gland

Accessory lacrimal gland

Lacrimal foramen and ducts

Lat. palpebral lig.

Sup. and inf. tarsi

Inf. rectus and oblique mus.

Infraorbital n.

Nasolacrimal duct and opening into inf. nasal meatus

Plate 29.
The Eye: Vision

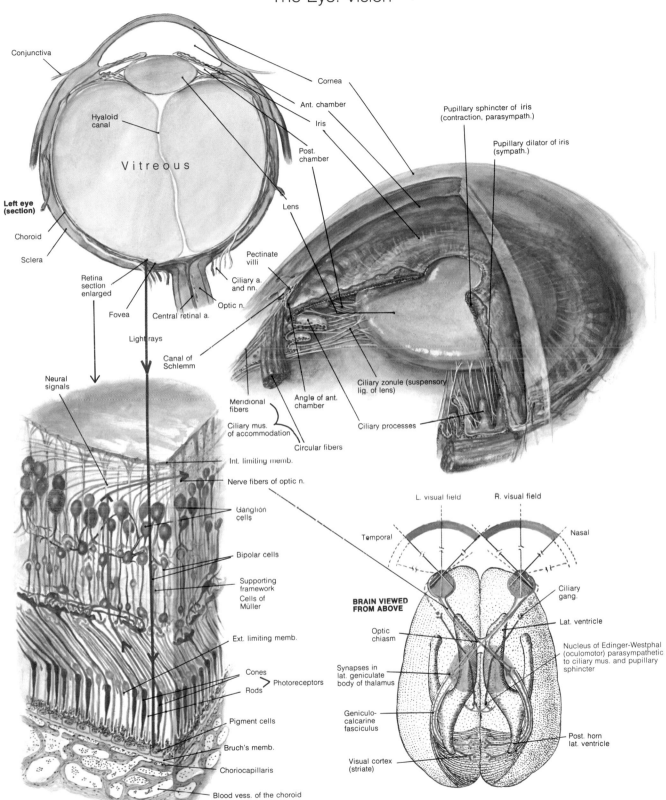

Conjunctiva

Hyaloid canal

Vitreous

Left eye (section)

Choroid

Sclera

Retina section enlarged

Fovea

Light rays

Neural signals

Cornea

Ant. chamber

Iris

Post. chamber

Lens

Pectinate villi

Ciliary a. and nn.

Optic n.

Central retinal a.

Canal of Schlemm

Meridional fibers

Angle of ant. chamber

Ciliary mus. of accommodation

Circular fibers

Pupillary sphincter of iris (contraction, parasympath.)

Pupillary dilator of iris (sympath.)

Ciliary zonule (suspensory lig. of lens)

Ciliary processes

Int. limiting memb.

Nerve fibers of optic n.

Ganglion cells

Bipolar cells

Supporting framework
Cells of Müller

Ext. limiting memb.

Cones
Rods } Photoreceptors

Pigment cells

Bruch's memb.

Choriocapillaris

Blood vess. of the choroid

L. visual field

R. visual field

Temporal

Nasal

BRAIN VIEWED FROM ABOVE

Optic chiasm

Synapses in lat. geniculate body of thalamus

Geniculo-calcarine fasciculus

Visual cortex (striate)

Ciliary gang.

Lat. ventricle

Nucleus of Edinger-Westphal (oculomotor) parasympathetic to ciliary mus. and pupillary sphincter

Post. horn lat. ventricle

The Ear

George T. Nager, M.D.

The ear may be divided into the external, middle, and inner portions. The external ear consists of the auricle, or pinna, and the external auditory canal. The auricle, which, in man, does little to increase the sensitivity of hearing, is made of a cartilaginous framework covered by skin, and is attached to the underlying temporal bone. Its sensory nerve supply is from the fifth, seventh, and tenth cranial nerves and from the cervical plexus.

The external auditory canal is bayonet-shaped and measures, in the adult, about 2.5 cm in length. It consists of an outer, cartilaginous portion and an inner, bony portion, and is lined with skin. In the cartilaginous portion the skin lining contains hairs and sebaceous and ceruminous glands.

The middle-ear cavity, except for its lateral wall, the tympanic membrane, is surrounded by bone and lined with mucous membrane. It communicates through the aditus with the mastoid and through the Eustachian tube with the nasopharynx. It contains the three middle-ear ossicles—malleus, incus, and stapes—which connect the tympanic membrane with the oval window and represent the normal pathway for sound transmission across the middle ear, which acts as a mechanical transformer. The muscles are attached to the ossicular chain. The tensor tympani muscle attaches to the neck of the malleus, and the stapedius muscle attaches to the neck of the stapes. These muscles represent a protective mechanism for the inner ear against very intense sound.

The Eustachian tube measures about 36 mm in length and consists of a lateral, bony portion and a medial, cartilaginous portion. Lined by respiratory epithelium and opening into the lateral wall of the nasopharynx, it provides exchange of air to the middle ear by the brief opening action of the tensor and levator muscles of the palate during swallowing.

Located in the petrous portion of the temporal bone, enclosed in the otic capsule, the inner ear houses the membranous cochlea and vestibular labyrinth, the sense organs of hearing and balance. The membranous cochlea and the vestibular labyrinth consist of a system of epithelial-formed spaces and tubes containing endolymph. This system is surrounded by the perilymph-filled periotic labyrinth, which in turn is enclosed in the bony labyrinth of the otic capsule. The perilymphatic system communicates through the cochlear aqueduct with the subarachnoid space. The endolymphatic system of the cochlea communicates with the saccular labyrinth through the ductus reuniens. The cochlea resembles a snail shell in appearance, with two and three-quarter turns in a horizontal plane, with its lower basal end forming the medial wall (promontory) of the middle ear. Each turn is made up of three compartments. The upper compartment of the cochlea, the scala vestibuli, is associated with the oval window, while the lower compartment, the scala tympani, ends at the round window. Both scalae are perilymph-filled and communicate at the apex, through the helicotrema. Between the two is the medial compartment, the scala media, or the cochlear duct. It extends from the cochlear recess of the vestibule to the cupular cecum at the apex of the cochlea. Near its basal end, the ductus reuniens provides communications of endolymph with the saccule. The cochlear duct, on a transverse section, has a triangular form. The floor of the cochlear duct is formed by the rigid basilar membrane; the lateral wall, by the stria vascularis of the spiral ligament: with the vestibular, or Reissner's, membrane forming the third wall.

The sensory receptors and supporting structures responsive to acoustic energy are located along the basilar membrane and form the organ of Corti. The organ of Corti contains a single row of 3,500 inner hair cells and three to four rows of over 20,000 outer hair cells. These hair cells are the sensory receptors to acoustic stimuli. The upper surface of the hair cells is formed by a thickened cuticular plate in which the stereocilia hairs are embedded in a specific pattern. The major support for the hair cells is provided at the superior surface, where they are attached to the rigid reticular lamina, which in turn is firmly attached to the basilar membrane by means of the pillar cells. The tectorial membrane, in which the stereocilia of the hair cells are embedded, on the other hand, has a loose attachment to the basilar membrane. Thus, displacement of the basilar membrane will differentially influence the cell bodies of the hair cells and the overlying tectorial membrane. Movement of the basilar membrane, by bending the stereocilia of the hair cells, initiates a transduction response in the sensory receptors. Beneath each hair cell, terminations of the afferent eight nerve fibers extend through the tunnel of Corti and enter the osseous spiral lamina. From there, they continue through Rosenthal's canal into the cochlear modiolus to join the main body of the cochlear nerve. Sound reaching the ear initiates a chain of mechanical and neural events that result in volleys of nerve impulses in the cochlear nerve. The volleys are relayed over afferent pathways to cell groups in the pons, midbrain, thalamus, and auditory receiving areas of the cortex.

The membranous vestibular labyrinth consists of the saccule, utricle, the three (superior, lateral, and posterior) semicircular canals, and the endolymphatic duct and sac. It is filled with endolymph and surrounded with perilymph. Both ends of each semicircular canal open into the utricle. Near the utricle, each canal enlarges to form the ampulla, which houses the crista, which is covered by a specialized neural epithelium. Two types of hair cells are found in this structure. The stereocilia of hairs of these cells insert into a gelatinous cupula, which extends from the surface of the crista to the roof of the ampulla. Displacement of endolymphatic fluid within the semicircular canal deviates the cupula relative to the surface of the crista, thus bending the hairs and initiating a transduction response in the sensory receptors. Each semicircular canal, which lies in a plane at a right angle to the other two, responds to angular acceleration (rotation) in its own plane. The utricle occupies the elliptical recess; the saccule, the spherical recess of the vestibule. Their sensory receptors and supporting structures form the maculae; in the saccule, the macula lies in a vertical plane, perpendicular to the macula of the utricle. The receptor cells in each are hair cells of two kinds, with kinocilia and stereocilia hairs projecting into an overlying otolithic membrane. Pressure changes on the underlying sensory receptors initiate the transducing response in these hair cells. Utricle and saccule are responsive to positional changes of the body, with the utricle being stimulated by centrifugal and vertical, and the saccule stimulated by linear, acceleration. The nerve fibers from the semicircular canals, utricle, and saccule join to form the vestibular portion of the eighth cranial nerve to reach the vestibular nuclei in the floor of the fourth ventricle. These nuclei have connections with the third, fourth, sixth, and tenth cranial nerves, with the spinal cord and with the cerebellar cortex.

Whereas the middle ear derives its blood supply mainly from branches of the external carotid artery, the inner ear is supplied by a branch of either the basilar or anterior inferior cerebellar artery of the vertebral system.

Plate 30.
The Ear: Apparatus of Hearing and Equilibrium

Auditory perception area (temporal gyrus)

Medial geniculate

Int. colliculus

Ext. auditory canal

R. EAR VIEWED FROM THE FRONT

Pons

Vestibular n., nuclei, and pathway to cerebellum for the regulation of equilibrium

Cochlear nuc.

Cochlear n.

Tympanic memb.

Semicircular canals

Cochlea

Inner ear

Middle ear

Reissner's memb.

Scala vestibuli

Bone

Stria vascularis

Scala media

Outer hair cells

Sensory receptors (sound)

Spiral lig.

Spiral prominence

Basilar memb.

Scala tympani

Inner hair cell

Cochlear n. fibers

Sup. semicircular canal

Membranous canal (contains endolymph)

Post. semicircular canal

Utricle

Endolymph. duct

Enlarged

Organ of Corti

Tectorial memb.

Bony canal (contains perilymph)

Crista sup. semicir. canal

Malleus

Ampulla lat. semicir. canal

Saccule

Sup. and int. vestibular gang.

Vestibular n.

Nervus intermedius

Facial n.

Lat. semicircular canal

Incus

Cochlear n.

Footplate of stapes in oval window

Scala tympani

Vestibule

Scala media

Promontory

Round window niche

Scala tympani

Scala media

Ductus reuniens

Perilymphatic duct

Helicotrema

Eustachian tube

Cochlea

Scala vestibuli

Scala media

The Nose, Paranasal Sinuses, Pharynx, and Larynx

Margaret M. Fletcher, M.D.

The nose represents the superiormost portion of the upper respiratory system. It plays an important part in the conditioning of the inspired air for the lower respiratory tract. This conditioning includes (1) the control of temperature, (2) the control of humidity, and (3) the elimination of dust and infectious organisms. Variation of outside temperature is considerable, ranging from plus 100 to minus 40 degrees Fahrenheit, but regardless of the outside level, the temperature of the inspired air is converted to about body temperature by the time it reaches the nasopharynx. This is achieved during its brief passage, about one-fourth of a second, through the nose, and is accomplished by the extensive capillary bed in the erectile tissue of the nasal turbinates. The rapid expansion and contraction of this tissue and its large vascular spaces with a rapid blood flow guarantee an instantaneous heat transfer from blood to air or vice versa. Similarly, the humidity of the outside air reveals a wide range, varying from less than 1 percent to more than 90 percent. By the time the inspired air reaches the nasopharynx, its relative humidity is converted to a constant 75 to 80 percent. The required rapid transfer of water from the nasal mucosa to the inspired air or vice versa is provided by the mucous blanket which covers the entire nasal mucosa.

The third important function of the nose is the active elimination of dust, infective organisms, and other particulate matter from the air before it reaches the nasopharynx. These particles are deposited on the mucous blanket. Constant ciliary action carries these particles to the nasopharynx and pharynx, from whence they drain into the stomach. The nasal secretions contain, among other substances, immunoglobulin or lysozyme, an enzyme that destroys bacteria on contact. Most organisms that enter the nose are destroyed in this manner. The rest are eliminated by the hydrochloric acid and other gastric secretions in the stomach. The mucous blanket in the nose travels approximately five to ten milimeters per minute. It is replaced about every twenty minutes from the submucosal glands and goblet cells. Thus, one of the several protective functions of the mucous blanket is to provide an effective defense mechanism against infections.

INTERNAL NOSE

The anterior nares open into a dilated portion of the nasal chamber called the *vestibule*. The vestibule is lined with skin that bears stiff hairs, which serve to filter large particles from the inspired air.

The surface area of the internal nasal chamber is doubled by the scroll-like projections on the lateral wall. These are the superior, middle, and inferior turbinates. Groovelike passages, called the *superior, middle,* and *inferior meatus,* exist between the turbinates. Beneath the inferior turbinate the nasal lacrimal duct enters the inferior meatus, 2 cm behind the mucocutaneous junction. The frontal, maxillary, and ethmoid sinuses open into the middle meatus beneath the middle turbinate.

OLFACTION

The olfactory epithelium covers the superior turbinate and adjacent nasal septum. Olfactory cells are bipolar neurons that are stimulated by lipid soluble substances in the inspired air. The axons penetrate the cribriform plate and synapse in the olfactory bulb. Secondary neurons then synapse in the central nervous system.

PARANASAL SINUSES

The paranasal sinuses are pneumatized areas in the frontal, maxillary, ethmoid, and sphenoid bone. They are lined with respiratory epithelium, which is continuous with that of the nasal cavity or upper airway. While the function of the paranasal sinuses is not

Plate 31.
The Nose and Paranasal Sinuses

Frontal sinuses and nasofrontal ducts

Sup. turbinate

Cartilages of ext. nose assure mobility and fracture resistance

Ethmoidal sinuses

Sphenoid sinuses and orifices

Lat. nasal cart.

Middle turbinate

Septal cart.

Maxillary sinuses and orifices

Sesamoid cart.

Minor alar cart.

Major alar cart. (lat. crus)

Inf. turbinate

Olfactory bulb and n. fibers

Post. ethmoidal a.

Nasal nn. and a.

Sphenopalatine gang. and a.

Ophthalmic a.

Palatine nn.

2nd cervical vert.

Pharyngeal orifice of Eustachian tube

Rosenmüller's fossa

Adenoid

Middle ethmoidal cells and orifices into middle meatus

Post. ethmoidal cells and orifices into sup. meatus

Sphenoid sinus and orifice

Clivus

L. frontal sinus

R. frontal sinus

Ant. ethmoidal a.

Bony framework of nose makes all portions of nasal fossa accessible to air currents in proper proportion. Deviation of air currents due to pathologic changes results in "jets" of inspired air which concentrate on mucosa. Infection may follow.

Ant. ethmoidal cells and orifices into infundibulum

Ethmoidal bulla

Hiatus semilunaris leading into infundibulum

Bony septum

Cartilaginous septum

Sup. meatus

Middle meatus

Inf. meatus

Maxillary sinus and orifice into nose

Nasolacrimal duct and orifice into inf. meatus

Uncinate process

Accessory orifice of maxillary sinus

Sup., middle, and inf. turbinates

Nasopalatine n. and vess.

Bony palate

Soft palate

Epiglottis

Vocal cords

entirely clear, they are important in the production of mucus and antibodies necessary for resistance to upper respiratory infections. They serve as resonating chambers and decrease the weight of the skull bones.

The frontal sinuses are located in the frontal bone. They are separated by a midline septum and extend laterally behind the superciliary arch and deeply over the orbit. The ethmoid sinuses are located between the eyes. They consist of a labyrinth of a number of air cells (3 to 18). Their boundaries are completed by the frontal, lacrimal, sphenoid, maxillary, and palatine bones. The ethmoid air cells open into the semilunar hiatus of the middle meatus.

The sphenoid sinus is important because of the company it keeps. It is bound laterally by the cavernous sinuses, which contain the carotid artery, third, fourth, fifth, and sixth cranial nerves. The superior boundary of the sphenoid sinus contains the optic canal, dura mater, and the pituitary gland. The sphenoid sinus empties into the sphenoethmoidal recess immediately lateral to the attachment of the nasal septum in the superior meatus.

The maxillary sinus is the largest of the paranasal sinuses. Its floor is formed by the alveolar process of the maxilla. A very thin plate of bone exists between the tooth roots and the sinus, a frequent source for infection. Laterally, the maxillary sinus extends into the zygomatic arch. The roof of the sinus is also the floor of the orbit.

PHARYNX

The pharynx serves as a common chamber for the respiratory and digestive tracts. It is divided into the nasal, oral, and laryngeal portions and is lined by respiratory epithelium superiorly and squamous epithelium inferiorly. It contains important lymphoid tissue for further protection of the human organism. The constrictor muscles of the pharyngeal wall are circular muscle fibers, which are important in swallowing.

NASOPHARYNX

The nasopharynx is bounded superiorly by the base of the skull and sphenoid rostrum, posteriorly by the cervical vertebrae, anteriorly by the posterior choana of the nose. The lateral walls contain the Eustachian tube orifices and the cartilagenous torus tubarius. Inferiorly it opens into the oral pharynx at the level of the soft palate. The Eustachian tube is important for ventilation of the middle ear, air being necessary in the middle ear in order to transmit sound through the ossicular chain. The pharyngeal tonsils on the posterior wall are important in the production of antibodies.

ORAL PHARYNX

From the level of the soft palate, the oral pharynx represents the digestive entrance of the chamber. The lateral walls are occupied by the palatine tonsils, which are bounded by the palatoglossal and palatopharyngeal folds. Inferiorly it extends to the level of the hyoid bone.

LARYNGEAL PHARYNX

The laryngeal pharynx lies behind the vestibule and posterior commissure of the larynx. Its anterior wall consists of the epiglottis, aryepiglottic folds, posterior commissure of the larynx, piriform sinuses laterally, and the posterior pharyngeal wall.

SWALLOWING REFLEX

A bolus of food is propelled posteriorly by the tongue. The nasopharynx is closed superiorly. As the food passes into the vallecula, the epiglottis folds over the laryngeal vestibule and the laryngeal muscles close reflexively. The cricopharyngeal muscle relaxes and the bolus of food enters the esophagus.

LARYNX

The larynx receives inspired air, which has been warmed, humidified, and filtered, and passes it on through the trachea and the bronchi to the lungs. The larynx acts as a valve to prevent the passage of foods and liquid into the area. There are nine laryngeal cartilages, which give the larynx a rigid form. Muscles act on the cartilages to modify the laryngeal aperture. The three single cartilages are the epiglottis, thyroid, and cricoid. The thyroid cartilage is composed of two lamina and provides support for the glottis. The strap muscles and inferior constrictor muscles of the pharynx are attached to the thyroid cartilage.

VOCAL APPARATUS

The form of the larynx is modified to control the expulsion of air from the lungs in order to produce sound. Paired arytenoid cartilages rotate on the cricoid cartilage to change the length and tension of the vocal cord for the production of sound.

The glottis is opened during inspiration by the posterior cricoarytenoid muscles. The glottis is closed during phonation and also to protect the airway by contraction of the lateral cricoarytenoid, transverse arytenoid, and the thyroarytenoid muscles.

Plate 32.
The Pharynx and Larynx

2nd cerv. vert.

Pharynx

Larynx

True cord

Trachea

Tracheal rings

Cricoid cart.

Thyroid cart.

Aryepiglottic lig.

Cuneiform cart.

Corniculate cart.

Transverse and
oblique arytenoid mus.

Recurrent
laryngeal n.
(motor)

Post. cricoarytenoid mus.

Vocal process
of arytenoid cart.

Laryngeal vent.

False cord

Thyroepiglottic lig.

Thyrohyoid memb.

Hyoid bone

Epiglottis

Soft palate

Hard palate

Sup. cornua

Thyroid
cart.

Cricothyroid
mus.

Cricoid cart.

Tracheal ring

Cricothyroid lig.

R. Lateral View

Anterior View

Int. br. sup. laryngeal n.
(sensory)

False cord
(ventricular
lig.)

True cord
(vocal lig.)

Apex of r.
arytenoid cart.

Ext. br. sup. laryngeal
a. (motor) to cricothyroid
and inf. constrictor mus.

R. arytenoid cart.

Lat. cricoarytenoid mus.

Muscular process of r.
arytenoid cart.

**VIEW FROM ABOVE
AND BEHIND**

Epiglottis (divided in midline)

Hyoid bone (divided in midline)

Aryepiglottic lig.

Cuneiform cart.

Corniculate cart.

Thyroid cart. (divided in midline)

Vocal process arytenoid cart.

Cricoid cart. divided
in midline

Transverse
arytenoid mus.

LATERAL VIEW

Vocal Apparatus

Sound is produced by vibrations
against edges of narrowed cord
opening (glottis) by air expelled
from lungs.

Arytenoid mus., which rotate arytenoid
cart. in a gliding motion upon rim of
cricoid cart., adjust size of glottic
opening (vent. and vocal lig.).

Attachment of
epiglottic lig.

Tongue

Laryngeal
ventricle

Cuneiform and
corniculate cart.

Epiglottis

False cord

True cord

Glottis

Quiet Respiration

MIRROR VIEW OF LARYNX

Wide Abduction

The Head and Neck

Melvin H. Epstein, M.D.
Donald S. Gann, M.D.
David W. Heese, D.D.S.
James J. Ryan, M.D.

The bones of the head consist of the cranium, encompassing the brain, and the bones of the facial skeleton. The facial bones are conveniently considered as bones of the midface—those of the orbit, nose, zygoma (cheek), and maxilla (upper jaw). The single bone of the lower face is the mandible, the only movable facial bone. The muscles associated with the midface are the muscles of facial expression, which, taking origin from the bones of the facial skeleton and attaching to the soft tissues of the eyelids, nose, cheeks, and lips, produce the facial movements of emotion and expression. These muscles are all innervated by the seventh cranial nerve. The muscles attached to the mandible, the muscles of mastication, arise from the cranium (i.e., the temporalis muscle) and the facial bones (i.e., the masseter muscle) and, with the tongue, form the floor of the mouth. These are all innervated by the fifth cranial nerve. In the neck the most prominent cervical muscle, the sternomastoid, divides the neck structures into anterior and posterior triangles.

BLOOD SUPPLY OF THE HEAD AND NECK

The scalp, face, and neck derive their blood supply primarily from the external carotid arteries. The external carotid is a terminal branch to the common carotid, which begins in the carotid triangle and passes upward and medial to the digastric muscle and the stylohyoid muscles. Eight branches arise from the external carotid artery. The superior thyroid artery arises at its lowest portion and terminates in the thyroid gland and the adjacent muscles and membranes attached to the thyroid cartilage. The lingual branch originates opposite the hyoid bone and ends beneath the tip of the tongue. The facial artery ends at the medial angle of the eye, where it anastomoses with the terminal branch of the ophthalmic artery. It provides the primary blood supply to the face, the tonsils, and the muscles at the base of the skull. The occipital branch supplies blood to the muscles of the back of the neck, in addition to the auricle and the posterior part of the scalp. There are meningeal branches that enter the skull and supply the dura mater. The posterior auricular branch ends near the mastoid process, behind the auricle. This artery supplies blood to the tympanic cavity, the antrum, the vestibule, the semicircular canals, and the mastoid air cells, as well as the scalp in the posterior temporal region.

The ascending pharyngeal artery supplies the wall of the pharynx and the soft palate. The superficial temporal artery, one of the terminal branches of the external carotid, has a small parotid branch and a small auricular branch, and the remaining branches give blood to the scalp, including the frontal belly of the occipitofrontalis and orbicularis oculi muscles. The maxillary artery is divided into three parts: the first part furnishes blood to the dura mater, the mandibular joint, the tympanic cavity, the mandible, teeth, and gingiva; the second part supplies the masseter muscle, the temporal muscle, and the buccal mucosa; and the third part furnishes blood to the orbit, the roof of the mouth, the gums and mucous membranes of the hard palate, the pharynx, the roof of the nose, the sphenoid sinus, and the ethmoid sinuses.

The vertebral artery is the first branch from the subclavian artery. It ascends, giving off muscular branches to the deep muscles of the neck and the suboccipital muscles, and ultimately enters the cranial cavity to supply the brain. The thyrocervical trunk, arising from the subclavian system, primarily supplies the muscles in the anterior part of the neck. The deep cervical artery also arises from the subclavian and primarily supplies the posterior muscles of the neck.

NERVE SUPPLY OF THE HEAD AND NECK

The anterior and posterior nerve roots divide into anterior and posterior primary rami, each of which are mixed sensory and motor nerves. The first cervical nerve is small. The posterior ramus supplies some of the muscles in the back of the neck, and the anterior primary ramus joins the hypoglossal nerve to supply the muscles attached to the larynx and hyoid bone. The posterior primary ramus of the second cervical nerve becomes the greater occipital nerve, the chief cutaneous nerve for the posterior part of the head. The posterior primary rami of the third, fourth, fifth, and sixth cervical nerves, small branches of minor importance, supply the skin of the back of the neck and some of the paraspinal muscles. The anterior primary rami of the first four cervical nerves form the cervical plexus. The cutaneous branches include the lesser occipital, greater auricular, and anterior cutaneous nerve from C2 and C3 roots, innervating the lateral skin of the neck and the scalp behind the ear. The supraclavicular nerves from the C3 and C4 root innervate the inferior lateral neck and the area of the chest several centimeters below the clavicle. There are muscular branches that arise from C2, C3, and C4 that innervate the sternomastoid, trapezius, and scalene muscles, and there are muscular branches that arise from C1 through C4 that innervate the prevertebral muscles and the diaphragm. There are also communicating branches that join the accessory nerve in its course to the trapezius muscle and communicating branches to the vagus nerve, hypoglossal nerve, and ansa hypoglossi.

The face is innervated by the fifth cranial nerve which is divided into three, the first division innervating the eye and some of the structures of the orbit, the second the cheek, and the third the chin. The nerve is discussed in detail in another section.

LYMPHATIC SYSTEM OF THE HEAD AND NECK

The lymphatic system of the head and neck converges principally about the jugular veins in the carotid sheaths, deep to the sternomastoid muscle. The superficial lymph nodes of the head (the occipital nodes, posterior auricular nodes, anterior auricular nodes, and superficial parotid nodes) drain into the superior deep cervical nodes. Likewise, the superficial lymph nodes of the neck (the submental and submaxillary nodes) have a similar drainage.

The deep lymph nodes of the neck are the retropharyngeal nodes medially, the juxtavisceral nodes (infrahyoid, prelaryngeal, pretracheal, and paratracheal nodes) anteriorly, and the superior medial and superior lateral nodes. All converge to drain into the supraclavicular nodes and thence down into the mediastinum. In addition to carrying lymphatic fluid from these regions, these nodes are active in body defenses against infection and cancer, in both of which states enlargement is common.

The other major glandular system of the head includes the major salivary glands. The largest of these, occupying the lateral cheek, is the parotid gland. In the floor of the mouth lie the small submaxillary glands and the smaller sublingual glands. These, in association with the innumerable minor salivary glands of the mouth, generate the salivary secretion commencing the digestive process. This varies greatly in volume, depending on digestive stimuli, but can amount to more than two liters daily.

THE ORAL CAVITY

The oral cavity is the beginning of the digestive tract. The bony support consists superiorly of the maxilla and inferiorly of the mobile mandible, attached by the temporomandibular joint. The cavity is divided into the vestibule, bounded medially by the teeth, and the cavity proper, bounded laterally and anteriorly by the teeth, posteriorly by the oral pharynx, superiorly by the hard and soft palate, and inferiorly by the attachment muscles of the tongue and the mylohyoid and genioglossus muscles.

Innervation of the oral cavity is supplied by the trigeminal nerve, whose branches are sensory to the teeth, mucous membranes, and anterior two-thirds of the tongue; and motor to the five muscles of mastication (masseter, temporalis, medial, and lateral pterygoid, and the anterior belly of the digastric). Other motor supply about the oral cavity comes from the facial nerve.

Blood supply to the oral cavity comes from various branches of the external carotid artery.

The lining of the area is mucous membrane, which contains many minor salivary glands. Surrounding the cavity and exiting into it are the major salivary glands: the parotid (Stensen's duct), the submaxillary (Wharton's duct), and the sublingual glands. These glands provide moisture for lubrication and add digestive enzymes, which begin the breakdown of the food.

Most of the cavity is filled by the highly muscular tongue, covered in the anterior two-thirds by hairy filiform and flat fungiform papillae. The posterior one-third is covered with the specialized circumvallate papillae. The tongue functions to move food to the

Plate 33.
Innervation of the Teeth and Facial Muscles; Salivary Glands and Muscles of Mastication

INNERVATION OF TEETH

Infraorbital n. emerging from infraorbital foramen

Ophthalmic n.

Maxillary n. and branches to teeth

Maxilla

Semilunar gang.

Greater palatine foramen and palatine nn. to soft palate

Mandibular n.

Ext. pterygoid mus. and n.

Pharyngopalatine arch

Int. pterygoid mus. and n.

Inf. alveolar n.

Inf. alveolar n.

Lingula

Lingual n.

Mandibular foramen

Glossopalatine arch

Mandible

Palatine tonsil

Muscles of mastication

Mental foramen

INNERVATION OF FACIAL MUSCLES OF EXPRESSION

Frontalis mus.

Orbicularis oculi mus.

Corrugator mus.

Temporal br.

Quadrate mus.

Zygomatic br.

Zygomatic mus.

Orbicularis oris mus.

Facial n.

Buccinator mus.

Buccal brs.

Triangularis mus.

Mandibular br.

Cervical br.

SALIVARY GLANDS AND MUSCLES OF MASTICATION

Temporalis mus.

Masseter mus.

Sublingual gland and openings of ducts (Rivinus')

Parotid gland and opening of duct (Stensen's)

Submaxillary gland and opening of duct (Wharton's)

grinding surfaces of the teeth and finally to deliver the bolus posteriorly to the oral pharynx and the esophagus. The oral pharynx is isolated from the nasal pharynx at this time by the lifting action of the soft palate.

The unique tissues in the mouth are the teeth, which are supported in the alveolar processes of the maxilla and mandible. In the adult dentition there are thirty-two teeth, divided into specialized tooth forms: the central and lateral incisors for cutting, the canines for tearing, the two premolars (bicuspids), and the three molars for grinding. Teeth are ectodermal (enamel) and mesodermal (dentin and pulp) in origin, and unlike most other body tissues are not capable of repair. Deciduous teeth are similarly named, but instead of premolars there are but two deciduous molars, which are replaced by premolars of the adult dentition. The permanent molars do not have deciduous predecessors.

THYROID AND PARATHYROID

The thyroid secretes hormones with diverse metabolic effects that act on nearly every tissue in the body. The thyroid follicles synthesize thyroxin (T4) and triiodothyronine (T3) from iodine and tyrosine. The uptake of iodide into the thyroid gland and its subsequent organification is under the control of the thyroid-stimulating hormone (TSH) from the anterior pituitary. TSH also controls release of a thyroid hormone in the bloodstream. Although both T4 and T3 are secreted, it is currently thought that most peripheral actions of the hormones occur through T3 following peripheral conversion from T4, the more slowly metabolized hormone. However, the feedback control of TSH release by the anterior pituitary operates through both T3 and T4. This feedback mechanism provides a control mechanism so that the principal mediator of release of TSH by the pituitary is the peripheral utilization of the thyroid hormones. The set point for this control system is provided by thyrotropin-releasing hormone (TRH) for the hypothalamus. This tripeptide provides a basis for some aspects of physiologic regulation. For example, cold leads to increased secretion of TRH. Most stresses, including surgery, decrease secretion of TSH, presumably through decreases in TRH. Although adrenal steriods also reduce TSH, this effect is also seen after adrenalectomy.

The thyroid hormones lead to increased oxygen consumption in most tissues except brain, spleen, and testes. The hormones lead directly to increased incorporation of amino acids into all tissues except for those named above, and lead to induction of a variety of enzymes. This induction of enzymes may be responsible for the increased metabolic rate seen with the hormones. Release of free fatty acids and glycogenolysis are enhanced by increased sensitivity to catecholamines. Finally, with the increased metabolic rate, the utilization of various coenzymes and vitamins is increased.

In addition, the C cells of the thyroid secrete a hormone, thyrocalcitonin, which is entirely independent of the system controlling T3 and T4. Secretion of thyrocalcitonin is stimulated by a rise in serum calcium and inhibited by a fall in the ion. This hormone thus participates, together with parathyroid hormone, in a double negative feedback system controlling serum calcium concentration. The hormone acts on bone to increase calcium uptake and bone formation and to decrease activity of osteoclasts. It also decreases renal excretion of calcium.

PARATHYROID

The parathyroid glands are the source of parathormone (PTH), which is the principal hormone controlling calcium metabolism. There are commonly four parathyroid glands, all of which receive their blood supply from branches of the inferior thyroid artery. The superior parathyroids may also receive branches from the superior thyroid arteries. In addition, the inferior parathyroid glands commonly lie anterior to the recurrent laryngeal nerve, whereas the superior parathyroid glands commonly lie posterior to this nerve. This relationship and the consistent arterial supply facilitate location of the parathyroid glands at surgery.

The major action of PTH is to increase serum calcium concentration by mobilizing calcium from bone. The action of the hormone appears to depend upon activation of cyclic AMP and perhaps on increased entry of magnesium ion into cells. In addition, osteoclastic activity is enhanced. PTH also acts upon the kidney to inhibit reabsorption of phosphate in the proximal tubule. The hormone also increases renal reabsorption of calcium, but because filtration of calcium is enhanced, there is a net increase in calcium excretion. Magnesium excretion is also enhanced, again because the filtered load is increased secondary to bone reabsorption. Finally, PTH acts upon the gut to increase absorption of calcium, but vitamin D is required for this effect.

Plate 34.
Sagittal Section of the Head and Neck; Thyroid and Parathyroid Glands

Parietal lobe
Choroid plexus
Sup. sagittal sinus
Third ventricle
Inf. sagittal sinus
Pineal gland
Septum pellucidum
Great cerebral v.
Corpus callosum
Aqueduct of Sylvius
Fornix
Straight sinus
Foramen of Monro
Occipital lobe
Frontal lobe
Cerebellum
Frontal sinus and opening of nasofrontal duct
Fourth ventricle
Ant. commissure
Pituitary gland
Optic chiasm
Pons
Sup., middle, and inf. turbinates
Basilar a.
Sphenoid sinus
Medulla oblongata
Bony palate
Dura
Tongue
Odontoid process—2nd cerv. vert.
Orifice of Eustachian tube
Soft palate
Hyoid bone
Spinal cord
Epiglottis
Thyroid cart.
Esophagus
False cord
Laryngeal ventricle
True cord
Trachea
Thyroid gland

MEDIAN SAGITTAL SECTION

Hyothyroid membrane
Int. carotid a.
Ext. carotid a.
Carotid sinus
Thyroid cart.
Int. jugular v.
Cricoid cart.
Cricoid cart.
Sup. thyroid vess.
Common carotid a.
Cricothyroid lig.
Post. cricoarytenoid mus.
Middle thyroid v.
Thyroid gland
Subclavian vess.
Parathyroid glands
Thyrocervical trunk
Inf. thyroid aa.
R. vagus n.
Inf. thyroid vv.
Recurrent laryngeal nn.
Aortic arch
Trachea
Lig. arteriosum
L. vagus n.

Anterior View

Posterior View

The Endocrine Glands

Donald S. Gann, M.D.

PITUITARY GLAND

The pituitary gland is attached to the median eminence of the hypothalamus. In addition to a direct arterial supply, the anterior lobe of this gland receives blood through a portal system from the hypothalamus. The activity of the posterior lobe is controlled directly by nerves with their cell bodies in supraoptic and paraventricular nuclei of the hypothalamus. This lobe secretes the hormones vasopressin and oxytocin. Secretion of vasopressin occurs in response to hypovolemia and to increased serum osmolality. Vasopressin increases reabsorption of water by the kidney by increasing permeability of the distal nephron. Increased secretion of oxytocin, which increases the letdown of milk and uterine tension, follows sucking or uterine distention.

Secretion of the hormones of the anterior pituitary gland is under the control of neurohormonal-stimulating and inhibiting factors released from the hypothalamus into the hypophysial portal vessels. The principal hormones include corticotropin (ACTH), melanophore-stimulating hormone, thyrotropin, prolactin, growth hormone, and gonadotropins. For each of these substances there appears to be a specific releasing hormone, and in some cases an inhibitory hormone as well. The principal pituitary hormones come from at least five different cell types in the human pituitary gland.

ACTH is released in response to all forms of stress, including pain, trauma, hemorrhage, fear, general sensory stimulation, cold, hypoglycemia, and immobilization. It exerts its principal effect on the zona fasciculata of the adrenal cortex to elicit secretion of cortisol. It also has a transient stimulating effect on secretion of aldosterone. In addition, ACTH acts independent of the adrenal to stimulate lipolysis.

Melanocyte-stimulating hormone (MSH) is a hormone that shares an amino acids sequence with amino acids 4 to 10 of ACTH. It is a major hormone in fish and amphibians, and functions in man to cause darkening of the skin. Little is known about its control. Its secretion is inhibited by MSH-inhibiting factor from the hypothalamus.

Growth hormone has a wide variety of metabolic effects. It increases incorporation of amino acids in muscle and liver and stimulates growth of cartilaginous epiphyses, which effects probably account for its growth-stimulating action. In addition, the hormone leads to retention of sodium, potassium, calcium, and phosphate by the kidney. Growth hormone has a transient lipogenic effect by increasing uptake of glucose into fat cells, but this gives way to a predominant lipolytic effect. In addition, growth hormone inhibits glucose entry into muscle cells and ultimately into fat cells, thus antagonizing the action of insulin. Gluconeogenesis is increased, adding further to the increase in concentration of glucose in blood.

The thyroid-stimulating hormone (TSH) acts on the thyroid gland to stimulate synthesis and secretion of the thyroid hormones thyroxin and triiodothyronine. Release of TSH is the result of an interaction between hypothalamic thyrotropin-releasing hormone (TRH), which stimulates release of TSH, and the feedback effects of thyroxin and triiodothyronine, which inhibit that release. In general the system acts to maintain a constant level of thyroid hormones in blood, so that its major drive is from peripheral utilization of hormone. Cold increases release of TRH, whereas general stress appears to decrease release of TRH.

Prolactin is a hormone that acts to maintain both lactation and the stability of the ovarian corpus luteum. Its secretion is controlled at least in part by TRH. There are some apparent interactions with circulating estrogens and progestins, but the mechanisms of control are not clear. In addition, there is some evidence that prolactin may be active in the control of renal handling of salt and water. Again, the physiologic mechanisms that may underlie this effect are obscure.

Follicle-stimulating hormone (FSH) facilitates the development of ovarian follicles and testicular tubules. Its secretion is controlled at least in part by circulating levels of gonadal steroids. Release of FSH is usually diminished after surgical stress.

Luteinizing hormone (LH) controls ovulation, the development of the corpus luteum, and, to some extent, estrogen secretion in the female, and stimulates secretion of testosterone in the male. Its release is inhibited by estrogen and by testosterone except under a priming condition, in which case the estrogen can facilitate the release of LH, bringing about a surge which leads to ovulation.

ADRENALS

The adrenal glands, as suggested by their name, lie above the kidneys bilaterally. They receive their arterial supply through end arteries that arise from phrenic, aortic, and renal vessels. In contrast, there is a central vein that collects all venous drainage from the adrenal cortex and medulla. The adrenal cortex consists of three zones and appears to be under humoral control. In contrast, the adrenal medulla consists of a single zone and is controlled primarily by the sympathetic nervous system.

The most external zone of the adrenal cortex, the zona glomerulosa, is responsible for secretion of aldosterone. This hormone controls, in part, the renal handling of salt and water. In the distal renal tubule it facilitates reabsorption of sodium chloride. In the late distal tubule and collecting duct it facilitates exchange of sodium for potassium and hydrogen and thus is the major factor controlling excretion of potassium and hydrogen. Secretion of aldosterone is controlled primarily by angiotensin II, formed in response to release of the enzyme renin by the kidney. Its secretion is also controlled by ACTH acutely and by the circulating level of potassium ion. The release of renin is controlled in a complex manner, but the cardiovascular baroreceptors and the sympathetic nervous system appear to play a dominant role.

The principal hormone secreted by the middle zone of the adrenal cortex, the zona fasciculata, is cortisol. Cortisol has a variety of metabolic effects. In all tissues except liver it inhibits incorporation of amino acids into cells. This leads to an antianabolic state and to net tissue catabolism. It may also be responsible for the anti-inflammatory action of this steroid, since lymphoid tissues are particularly sensitive to its action. In the liver cortisol facilitates the uptake of amino acids and stimulates both gluconeogenesis and albumin synthesis. In all cells cortisol inhibits the uptake of glucose. These effects lead to a net increase in serum glucose concentration. In addition, the hormone facilitates the movement of potassium and water from cells into the extracellular space. Except for the immediate action on glucose uptake, most of the actions of the steroid appear to involve incorporation of the hormone into the nucleus and formation of mRNA. The control of cortisol secretion is almost exclusively by pituitary ACTH.

The zona reticularis of the adrenal gland, the inner cortical zone, is responsible for adrenal secretion of androgens and estrogens. This zone is primarily controlled by ACTH, although FSH or other pituitary factors may also play a role. Substantial amounts of sex steroids may be of adrenal origin.

The adrenal medulla is controlled primarily by the sympathetic nervous system. The transmitter is acetylcholine, released by sympathetic nerve endings and stimulating directly synthesis and release of epinephrine and norepinephrine. These hormones act to stimulate α and β receptors, leading to peripheral vasoconstriction, increased myocardial contractility, glycogenolysis, lipolysis, and a multitude of other effects. The release of catecholamines by the adrenal medulla is also facilitated by angiotensin II, so that there is a positive feedback mechanism relating these two factors. Finally, the synthesis of epinephrine requires the adrenal cortical hormone cortisol.

PANCREAS

The endocrine functions of the pancreas are based in the islands of Langerhans. These islands are distributed throughout the pancreatic tissue but concentrated somewhat in the tail of the pancreas. The principal functions of the island cells are secretion of insulin (β-cell) and of glucagon (α-cell). Insulin facilitates glucose transport into cells together with potassium, increases glycogenesis, and lowers blood concentration of glucose. In addition, insulin acts on muscle to increase incorporation of amino acids and to increase formation of protein. Insulin also acts on fat cells to increase glucose entry and oxidation and to lead to lipogenesis. Insulin does not affect glucose entry into liver cells but does increase glycogen formation, decrease glycolytic activity, and induce glucose-6-phosphate dehydrogenase activity. Secretion of insulin is stimulated by an increase in plasma glucose and by parasympathetic nervous activity, and is inhibited by sympathetic nervous activity and by epinephrine.

Plate 35.
Endocrine Glands

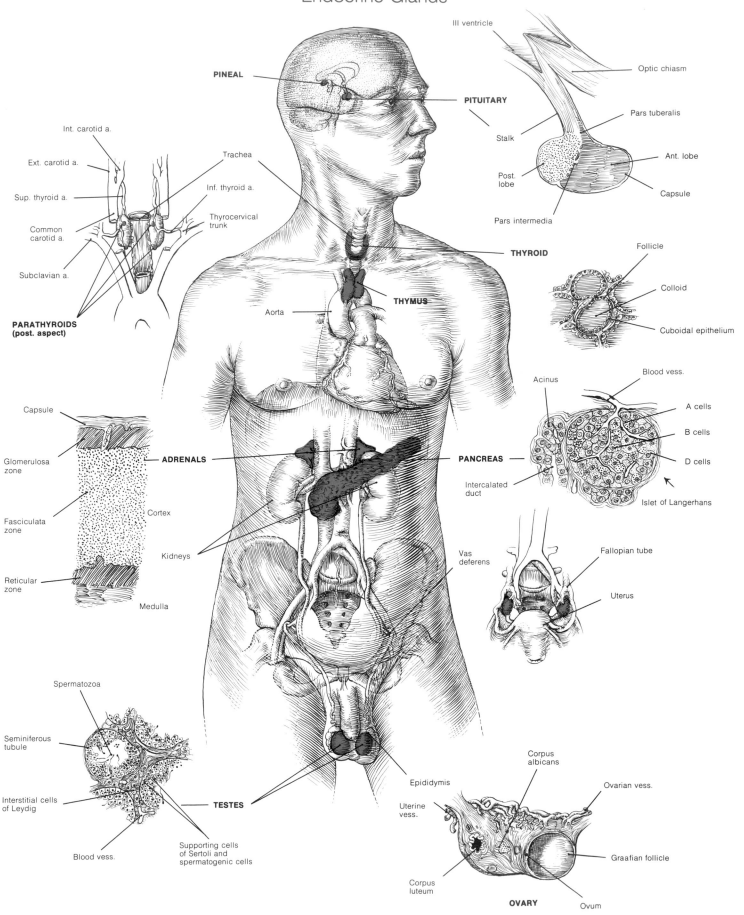

III ventricle

PINEAL

PITUITARY

Optic chiasm

Stalk

Pars tuberalis

Post. lobe

Ant. lobe

Pars intermedia

Capsule

Int. carotid a.

Ext. carotid a.

Sup. thyroid a.

Common carotid a.

Subclavian a.

Trachea

Inf. thyroid a.

Thyrocervical trunk

THYROID

Follicle

Colloid

Cuboidal epithelium

PARATHYROIDS (post. aspect)

Aorta

THYMUS

Acinus

Blood vess.

A cells

B cells

D cells

Capsule

Glomerulosa zone

Fasciculata zone

Reticular zone

Medulla

ADRENALS

Cortex

Kidneys

PANCREAS

Intercalated duct

Islet of Langerhans

Vas deferens

Fallopian tube

Uterus

Spermatozoa

Seminiferous tubule

Interstitial cells of Leydig

Blood vess.

TESTES

Supporting cells of Sertoli and spermatogenic cells

Epididymis

Corpus albicans

Uterine vess.

Ovarian vess.

Graafian follicle

Corpus luteum

OVARY

Ovum

Plate 36.
Physiology of Endocrine Glands
(Schematic Summary)

PHYSIOLOGICAL STIMULI	GLAND	HORMONE	TARGET ACTIVITY
VOLUME, TONICITY	POST. PIT.	VASOPRESSIN	ANTIDIURESIS, VASOCONSTRICTION
UTERINE DISTENTION	POST. PIT.	OXYTOCIN	UTERINE CONTRACTION, MILK EJEC.
HYPOGLYCEMIA	ANT. PIT.	GROWTH HORMONE	VARIOUS METABOLIC EFFECTS, SOMATIC GROWTH
?	ANT. PIT.	PROLACTIN	MAINTAINS CORPUS LUTEUM—LACTATION
?	ANT. PIT.	FSH	FOLLICLE GROWTH, SPERMATOGENESIS. OVULATION. ESTROGEN, PROGESTERONE
?	ANT. PIT.	LH	TESTOSTERONE
DECREASED METAB. RATE, COLD	ANT. PIT.	THYROTROPIN	INCREASED THYROID SECRETION
STRESSES	ANT. PIT.	CORTICOTROPIN (ACTH)	INCREASED ADRENAL CORTICAL SECRETION, LIPOLYSIS
STRESSES (ACTH)	ADRENAL CORTEX	CORTISOL	GENERAL METABOLIC EFFECTS
HYPOVOLEMIA, HYPERKALEMIA	ADRENAL CORTEX	ALDOSTERONE	SALT RETENTION, K⁻ LOSS
STRESSES (SYMPATHETIC)	ADRENAL MEDULLA	EPINEPHRINE—NOREPINEPHRINE	GLYCOGENOLYSIS, α & β ADRENERGIC ACTIONS
HYPERGLYCEMIA	PANCREAS β	INSULIN	GENERAL METABOLIC EFFECT
HYPOGLYCEMIA	PANCREAS α	GLUCAGON	
INCREASED METABOLIC RATE (TSH)	THYROID	THYROXIN, T3	INCREASED METABOLISM
INCREASED CALCIUM	THYROID	THYROCALCITONIN	DECREASED CALCIUM
DECREASED CALCIUM	PARATHYROID	PARATHORMONE	INCREASED CALCIUM
LH	OVARY	ESTROGEN	PROTEIN ANABOLISM, SEX ORGANS
LH	OVARY	PROGESTERONE	ENDOMETRIAL PROLIFERATION
LH	TESTIS	TESTOSTERONE	PROTEIN ANABOLISM, SEX ORGANS
NOT IDENTIFIED POSITIVELY	THYMUS	NOT KNOWN	LYMPHOCYTE STIMULATION

Glucagon increases glycogen breakdown and glycogenolysis in the liver but stimulates glucose uptake into muscle. It stimulates lipolysis but lowers plasma fatty acids, probably by increasing uptake into liver and muscle. It inhibits amino acid incorporation into muscle. In addition, this hormone decreases serum calcium and increases cardiac contractility. Secretion of glucagon is stimulated by hypoglycemia and by sympathetic nervous activity and inhibited by parasympathetic nervous activity.

THYROID

The thyroid gland is formed of two lobes, which lie over the trachea in the neck. Its principal secretory products are thyroxin and triiodothyronine, which regulate metabolism primarily through induction of enzymes. These hormones act at a number of sites synergestically with the catecholamines. In addition, both hormones act on the pituitary gland to inhibit release of TSH, which in turn stimulates the secretion of thyroid hormones. The thyroid also secretes thyrocalcitonin, which increases calcium incorporation into bone and decreases calcium excretion by the kidney. Secretion of this hormone is stimulated by hypercalcemia, and its net effect is to decrease the level of serum calcium in blood.

PARATHYROIDS

The parathyroid glands usually number four and are located on either side adjacent to the thyroid gland. Parathormone, the principal secretory product, acts to mobilize calcium from bone, increase gut absorption of calcium, and increase renal excretion of phosphate. These effects interact to increase the serum concentration of calcium and decrease the serum concentration of phosphate. Parathormone secretion is stimulated by hypocalcemia and inhibited by hypercalcemia.

TESTES

The principal secretory product of the testes is testosterone. This hormone is secreted by the interstitial cells in response to pituitary luteinizing hormone (LH). Testosterone acts to produce virilization and to increase amino acid incorporation into muscle, liver, and kidney. Bone growth is accelerated, but terminates when the epiphyses close in response to the action of the hormone. Red cell production is also stimulated. Some estrogen is also secreted by the testes in response to the action of FSH and LH.

THYMUS

The thymus lies in the anterior mediastinum anterior to the trachea. No specific hormones have been identified, but there appear to be one or more thymic hormones. The thymus appears to inhibit production of cells of the anterior pituitary that synthesize growth hormone, whereas growth hormone in turn increases thymic size. In addition, a thymic factor increases the number of stem cells in bone marrow. There is also evidence for a lymphocytosis-stimulating factor and for a factor that induces immunocompetence. In addition, a factor has been identified that inhibits neuromuscular transmission. Whether these effects are the result of actions of a single hormone or of multiple hormones is not known.

15

The Circulatory System

Robert K. Brawley, M.D.

The circulatory system consists of the heart, a pump (described in the next chapter), and the blood vessels, a network of tubes that carry blood to and from the heart (Plate 37). Blood vessels are designated arteries, arterioles, capillaries, or veins depending upon their size, composition, and function. Arteries vary in size from large, named vessels to very small and unnamed vessels, but all carry blood from the heart to the body tissues. The walls of the arteries contain three layers; adventitia (outer layer), media, and intima (inner layer). The media of the larger arteries (aorta, innominate, subclavian) contains large amounts of elastic tissue and few smooth muscle cells, while the media of the medium-sized arteries (radial, popliteal, superior mesenteric) and the smaller, unnamed arteries have many smooth muscle cells and relatively little elastic tissue. Smooth muscle cells are particularly prominent in the walls of the arterioles, which are extremely small vessels about 0.2 mm in diameter and just visible without magnification.

The smooth muscle cells of the arteries and the arterioles are innervated by autonomic nerves. Impulses from the sympathetic nerves cause the smooth muscle to contract, thus diminishing the vessel diameter, while impulses from parasympathetic nerves produce smooth muscle relaxation and result in dilatation of the vessels; blood flow to various regions of the body is regulated in this way. The coronary arteries are exceptions to this rule, since in these vessels sympathetic impulses cause dilatation and parasympathetic impulses produce constriction. Arterioles lead into capillaries, vessels approximately 1 mm long that have a lumen about the diameter of a red blood cell (7 to 8 microns). The capillary wall consists of a single layer of endothelial cells, which permits exchange of oxygen, carbon dioxide, nutrients, and waste products between the body tissues and the blood. Veins carry blood from the capillaries to the heart. Usually, veins have the same name as the adjacent artery. Although vein walls have the same three layers as arteries, the media of the veins is poorly developed, and thus the walls of veins are less thick than the walls of arteries of similar diameter.

The aorta is the main trunk of the systemic arterial system, and its parts are designated the ascending aorta, the arch of the aorta, and the thoracic and abdominal portions of the descending aorta (Plate 38). The ascending aorta, located in the middle mediastinum, begins at the aortic valve and ends at the innominate artery (brachiocephalic trunk). Its only branches are the left and right coronary arteries. The arch of the aorta lies in the superior mediastinum and has three branches; the innominate artery, the left common carotid artery, and the left subclavian artery. After a short distance, the innominate artery divides into the right subclavian and right common carotid arteries. The arteries that provide the major portion of blood supply to the head and neck are the right and left common carotid arteries, each of which divides into two branches: the external carotid, supplying the neck, the face, and the exterior of the head; and the internal carotid artery, supplying the anterior brain, eye, orbit, and sinuses. The subclavian artery brings blood to the upper extremities. It becomes the axillary artery at the lower border of the first rib, and at the lower border of the axilla it becomes, in turn, the brachial artery, which divides into the radial and ulnar arteries at the elbow. Branches of the subclavian artery include the vertebral and the internal mammary arteries (internal thoracic artery).

The descending thoracic aorta traverses the posterior mediastinum and gives rise to intercostal, bronchial, esophageal, pericardial, mediastinal, and diaphragmatic branches. The intercostal arteries course below each rib and form anastomoses with the intercostal branches of the internal mammary arteries. Blood is supplied to the spinal cord principally by the anterior spinal artery but also by the two posterior spinal arteries (Plate 38). The anterior spinal artery is formed at the level of the medulla oblongata from branches of the two vertebral arteries. This artery descends along the anterior aspect of the spinal cord and gives off numerous circumferential and penetrating branches, which provide the blood supply to the spinal cord itself. The posterior spinal arteries take origin from the cerebellar arteries and descend along the posterior aspect of the spinal cord. They also send penetrating branches into the spinal cord. These three spinal arteries are joined at numerous sites along their courses by radicular spinal branches of the vertebral, cervical, intercostal, lumbar, and sacral segmental arteries (Plate 38). Of specific interest is the artery of Adamkiewicz, which is a relatively large radicular spinal branch of the lower intercostal or upper lumbar arteries. The artery of Adamkiewicz connects with the anterior spinal artery in the vicinity of the crura of the diaphragm and provides important blood supply to the spinal cord. Interruption of the posterior spinal arteries may produce no untoward effect because of extensive anastomoses. However, interruption of the anterior spinal artery or the artery of Adamkiewicz will often result in paralysis.

As the aorta passes through the aortic hiatus of the diaphragm, it is designated the abdominal portion of the descending aorta, or, more simply, the abdominal aorta. The first branches of the abdominal aorta are the phrenic arteries, which supply the inferior surface of the diaphragm. The celiac artery arises from the aorta just below the aortic hiatus and has three major branches: the common hepatic artery, the splenic artery, and the left gastric artery. As their names imply, these branches provide blood supply to the liver, the spleen, and a major portion of the stomach. In addition, much of the duodenum and pancreas receive blood from branches of these arteries. The superior mesenteric artery arises from the aorta about 1 cm below the celiac artery and supplies the entire small intestine except for the proximal duodenum; it also gives blood supply to the cecum, the ascending colon, and the proximal one-half of the transverse colon. The renal arteries take origin from the aorta just distal to the superior mesenteric arteries. The abdominal aorta also gives origin to the suprarenal, testicular, or ovarian arteries and four pairs of lumbar arteries. The lumbar arteries supply blood to the lateral and posterior abdominal walls and to the spinal cord via spinal branches. The inferior mesenteric artery takes origin from the abdominal aorta about 3 or 4 cm above the aortic bifurcation, and supplies the distal one-half of the transverse colon, the descending colon, the sigmoid colon, and a major part of the rectum. At the level of the fourth lumbar vertebra the abdominal aorta bifurcates into the left and right common iliac arteries. The middle sacral artery, a small vessel, arises from the posterior wall of the aorta just proximal to its bifurcation. The common iliac arteries divide to form the internal and external iliac arteries. The internal iliac, or hypogastric, artery supplies structures of the pelvis, the buttock, the generative organs, and the medial aspect of the thigh. The external iliac artery passes along the wall of the pelvis and at the inguinal ligament becomes the common femoral artery, which is the major source of blood supply for the lower extremity. The femoral triangle is a space formed by the inguinal ligament and the border of the sartorius and adductor longus muscles and through which course the femoral artery, vein, and nerve. The common femoral artery divides into the superficial femoral artery and the deep femoral, or profunda femoris, artery about 3 cm below the inguinal ligament. This latter artery is a major source of blood supply to the structures of the thigh. The superficial femoral artery traverses Hunter's canal in the thigh and becomes the popliteal artery at the knee. Below the knee, the popliteal artery divides into three branches: the anterior tibial artery, the posterior tibial artery, and the peroneal artery. These arteries supply the lower leg and the foot.

The superior vena cava is the great vein that receives blood from the upper body and returns it to the heart; the inferior vena cava serves the same function for the lower part of the body. The internal jugular veins receive blood from the brain, face, and neck, while the subclavian veins collect blood from the upper extremities. The internal jugular and the subclavian veins join to form the innominate (brachiocephalic) veins, which, in turn, join to form the superior vena cava.

The veins of both the upper and lower extremities are classified as either deep or superficial, depending upon their position relative to the deep fascia of the extremity. In the lower extremity, the superficial venous system consists of the long and short saphenous veins and their tributaries (Plate 39). The long and short saphenous veins connect with one another through several communicating veins. The deep venous system is composed of the popliteal and femoral veins and their tributaries. The superficial and deep venous systems communicate at the knee where the short saphenous vein passes through the popliteal fascia to enter the popliteal vein and at the groin where the long saphenous vein joins the femoral vein by penetrating the fascia at the fossa ovalis. In addition to these two principal sites of

Sup. long. sinus
Ascending cerebral
Lat. sinus
Int. jugular
Vertebral
Subclavian
Innominate
R. innominate
L. innominate
Axillary
Sup. vena cava
Cephalic
R. pulm.
Brachials
Sinuses of Valsalva
R. coronary
Hepatic
Suprarenal
Gastroduodenal
Median basilic
Renals
Sup. mesenteric
Middle colic
R. colic
Spermatic
Ileocolic
Common iliacs
Cephalic
Ext. iliac
Int. iliac
Basilic
Median
Sup. hemorrhoidal
Obturator
Inf. gluteal
Femoral
Int. pudendal
Greater saphenous
Popliteal
Med. circumflex
Lesser saphenous
Greater saphenous
Post. tibial

Pericallosal
Callosomarginal
Frontopolar
Ant. cerebral
Middle cerebral
Sup. temporal
Maxillary
Post. auricular
Occipital
Facial
Int. carotid
Ext. carotid
Lingual
Sup. thyroid
Trans. scapular and sup. cervical
Inf. thyroid
Axillary
Thyrocervical trunk
Thoracoacromial
Lat. thoracic
Subscapular
L. common carotid
L. subclavian
Int. mammary
Brachial
Profunda brachii
L. pulm.
Circumflex
L. coronary
L. gastric
L. ant. descending coronary
Splenic
Celiac
Int. mesenteric
Recurrent
L. colic
Radial
Interosseous
Pancreatico duodenal
R. gastroepiploic
Middle colic
Ulnar
Middle sacral
Iliolumbar
Deep circumflex iliac
Lat. circumflex
Inf. epigastric
Common femoral
Profunda femoris
Sup. gluteal
Sup. femoral
Popliteal
Ant. tibial
Peroneal
Dorsalis pedis
Lat. plantar
Med. plantar

Ao.

Sup. volar arch
Deep volar arch

Post. communicating
Post. cerebral
Basilar
Ophthalmic
Vertebral

Portal
L. branch portal
Pyloric
Cystic
R. branch portal
Esophageal
Coronary
Short gastrics

Liver

Spleen
L. gastroepiploic
Splenic
L. colic
Inf. mesenteric
Iliocolic
R. colic
Sup. mesenteric

SPLENOPORTAL SYSTEM

Red = arteries
Gray = veins

Plate 38.
The Aorta and Branches

R. common carotid a.

Thyro-cervical trunk

Innominate a.

Ascending aorta

R. bronchial a.

Descending aorta

L. and r. coronary aa.

Diaphragm

Aortic hiatus of diaph.

Celiac a.

Sup. mesenteric a.

Renal aa.

Testicular or
ovarian aa.

Inf. mesenteric a.

Common iliac aa.

Middle sacral a.

Int. iliac a.
(hypogastric)

Lat. sacral a.

Obturator a.

Inf. epigastric a.

Inf. gluteal a.

Inf. pudendal a.

Superficial ext.
pudendal a.

Deep ext. pudendal a.

Adductor longus mus.

Adductor canal
(Hunter's)

Vastus medialis mus.

Popliteal a.

Post. tibial a.

Peroneal a.

L. common carotid a.

Vertebral a.

L. subclavian a.

Clavicle

Int. mammary a.
(int. thoracic)

1st intercostal a.

L. bronchial aa.

Thoracic
intercostal aa. (9)

Lumbar aa. (5)

Iliolumbar a.

Ext. iliac a.

Sup. gluteal a.

Deep circumflex a.

Inguinal lig.

Sartorius mus.

Lat. femoral
circumflex a.

Femoral canal

Femoral v., a., and n.
(femoral triangle)

Pectineus mus.

Deep femoral a.

Sup. femoral
and v.

Saphenous n.

Ant. tibial a.

Basilar a.

Vertebral aa.

Medulla oblongata

1st cervical n.

Ant. spinal a.

1st thoracic a.

**Anterior View
of Spinal Cord**

Radicular spinal branches
from intercostal aa.

12th thoracic n.

Conus medullaris
(end of spinal cord)

Ant. spinal a.

1st lumbar
vert.

1st lumbar n.

Lumbar sacral and
coccygeal nn.

Sacrospinalis mus.

Spinal cord

Post. spinal a.

Post. ramus

Ant. ramus
(intercostal)

Artery of Adamkiewiez
(spinal branch)

Spinal branch

Sympathetic chain

Thoracic
intercostal aa.

Aorta

**CROSS SECTION AT
LEVEL OF TENTH
THORACIC VERTEBRA**

Plate 39.
Muscular Venous Pump of Leg

Popliteal v.

Post. tibial venae comitantes

Crural fascia

Lesser saphenous v.

Greater saphenous v.

Dorsal venous arch

Valves

Perforating v. penetrating crural fascia

Communicating vv.

Calcaneal tendon

RELAXED MUSCULAR VENOUS PUMP

DILATED VEINS

SOLEUS AND GASTROCNEMIUS MUSCLES

VENOUS AND LYMPHATIC FLOW TOWARD HEART

Open Valve
permits venous blood flow to heart (antegrade)

Closed Valve
prevents venous blood from flowing backward (retrograde)

Aerolar tissue

Lymphatics

Veins

Compressed lymphatics

Magnified representation

Muscle bundle

Propulsion of blood (veins) and tissue fluid (lymphatics) toward heart

COMPRESSED VEINS WITHIN MUSCLE CONTAINED WITHIN CRURAL FASCIA

Fibula

Tibia

CONTRACTED MUSCULAR-VENOUS PUMP

Strong crural fascial compartments aid in compression of veins

Crural fascia

Gastrocnemius mus. (tendon)

Soleus mus. (tendon)

Calcaneal tendon

TO RELAX PUMP

TO CONTRACT PUMP (WALKING)

communication, the superficial and deep systems are connected at numerous points by unnamed perforating veins that pierce the fascia of the leg. Both superficial and deep veins of the lower extremities contain numerous valves. The femoral veins receive tributary veins from the lower extremities and, as they pass under the inguinal ligaments, become the iliac veins, which also collect blood from the pelvic structures. The right and left common iliac veins join to form the inferior vena cava, which, as it traverses the abdominal cavity, is joined by the right spermatic or ovarian vein, renal veins, suprarenal veins, hepatic veins, and lumbar veins. The portal vein is formed by the merging of the superior mesenteric and splenic veins, which receive blood from intestines, pancreas, and spleen (Plate 37, insert). Blood from the portal vein passes through the liver and is collected by the hepatic veins, which join the inferior vena cava just below the diaphragm.

The function of the circulatory system is to provide blood flow that brings oxygen and nutrients to and carries carbon dioxide and waste products away from peripheral tissues. A region of the body is said to be ischemic when blood flow to that area is inadequate to allow normal function. In the presence of severe ischemia, cellular metabolism, which is usually aerobic, becomes anaerobic. Carbon dioxide and lactic acid accumulate, and metabolic acidosis develops in the region. When cardiac output (the amount of blood pumped by the heart into the arteries each minute) becomes abnormally low, the body alters the distribution of blood flow and shunts blood to more vital body areas, such as the heart and brain, and away from the musculoskeletal and splanchnic vascular beds. This shunting of blood is accomplished, in part through the autonomic nervous system by constricting or dilating arteries, particularly arterioles, thereby changing resistance to blood flow in various body regions.

As the blood is pumped through the arteries by the heart and as it returns to the heart through the veins, it exerts a certain pressure within the blood vessels. Arterial blood pressure is a product of the cardiac output and the peripheral resistance to blood flow that exists in the arterial system at any given moment. Cardiac output is largely determined by the adequacy of the heart as a pump and by the blood volume. Resistance is primarily a function of the status of the arterioles, but it is also influenced by the diameter of the muscular arteries, the elasticity of the larger arteries, and viscosity of the blood. Hemorrhage that seriously depletes blood volume and myocardial damage that diminishes the power of the heart can result in decreased cardiac output and an abnormally low blood pressure, i.e., hypotension or shock. A variety of pathologic conditions can cause increased peripheral resistance due to severe constriction of arterioles and produce abnormally high blood pressure, i.e., hypertension.

Once the blood passes through the capillaries, most of the energy of cardiac contraction has been expended to overcome the resistance of the arterioles and capillary beds. In the supine subject, a small pressure gradient exits between the peripheral veins and the right atrium and propels blood toward the heart. In the erect position, the force of gravity acts to retard venous return to the heart from the lower extremities, and the "pumping" mechanism of the muscles of the legs and the existence of valves in the veins of the extremities become important factors in preventing stasis of blood in the venous system (Plate 39). Thrombophlebitis can destroy the valves of the veins and result in venous stasis, varicose veins, and skin ulcers. During walking the gastrocnemius and soleus muscles contract, thereby increasing pressure in the veins and lymphatics of the calf. The increased pressure tends to propel blood in the veins and tissue fluids in the lymphatics toward the heart. As the muscles of the leg relax, pressure in the veins diminishes and blood in the veins begins to flow toward the feet. This retrograde blood flow is prevented by the venous valves, which close and hold the blood in that segment of vein until the next muscular contraction again forces blood antegrade toward the heart. Soldiers standing at attention for long periods of time are known to be susceptible to fainting due to pooling of blood in their lower extremities. They are usually advised to tighten their calf muscles periodically to help move blood from legs to the heart.

The Heart

Vincent L. Gott, M.D.

CARDIAC STRUCTURES AND FUNCTION

The adult human heart, weighing approximately 300 grams, is an extremely efficient muscular pump, designed to contract 42 million times a year and eject 700,000 gallons of blood during the same period. Although the design of this muscular pump is relatively simple from the standpoint of mechanical structure, the control mechanism for heart rate and cardiac output is exquisitely sensitive and thus quite elaborate.

The right atrium serves as the receiving chamber for all the systemic venous blood returning through the superior and inferior venae cavae. During the period of cardiac relaxation (ventricular diastole), blood flows from the right atrium into the right ventricle, and then, during ventricular systole, this blood is ejected through the pulmonary valve into the pulmonary circulation. The two valves (tricuspid valve and pulmonary valve) serve simply to permit a one-way flow of blood in an efficient manner through the right heart and into the pulmonary vasculature. In the normal heart, the pressure rises to approximately 5 mm Hg in the right atrium during contraction of this chamber. Pressure within the right ventricle is normally 25/0 (systole/diastole). Since there is no perceptible gradient across any of the normal heart valves, pressure in the pulmonary artery is normally 25/10.

Oxygenated blood returns from the lungs to the left atrium through the pulmonary veins and then, during ventricular diastole, flows through the mitral valve and into the left ventricle. Again, during ventricular systole, blood is ejected by the left ventricle into the ascending aorta through the aortic valve. The aortic valve is very similar in appearance to the pulmonary valve in that it has three delicate cusps, or pockets, which again permit blood flow in only one direction. The tricuspid and mitral valves, on the other hand, have leaflets tethered by fibrous cords (chordae tendineae) attached to the papillary muscles in the apex of each of the two ventricles. The tricuspid valve, of course, has three separate cusps, and the mitral valve has two leaflets.

Normal pressure in the left atrium during atrial contraction is approximately 15 mm Hg, and, during left ventricular contraction, the pressure in this latter chamber rises to approximately 120 mm Hg, with a similar systolic pressure in the ascending aorta. Ordinarily, the period of systole takes less than 0.3 second and the period of diastole is approximately 0.7 second. During diastole, pressure in the aorta falls to a level of approximately 80 mm Hg.

The right and left coronary arteries arise from the root of the aorta, with the orifices of each of these vessels being situated in the sinuses of the aortic valve. The left coronary artery courses behind the pulmonary artery and divides within 2 cm into the anterior descending artery and the circumflex artery. The right coronary artery courses on the surface of the heart between the right atrium and the right ventricle, and its blood supply terminates in the diaphragmatic surface of the heart. After coronary blood passes through the capillaries of the myocardium, approximately 60 percent of venous flow enters the right atrium through the large coronary sinus vein, and the remaining flow drains into the left atrium and the left and right ventricles through the Thebesian veins. Unlike in any other organ in the body, the greatest flow of blood takes place through the heart during the period of diastole. During the ejection phase of ventricular systole, coronary blood flow is greatly reduced because of compression of the coronary vessels by the cardiac muscle fibers.

All of the structures of the heart, of course, can be affected by disease or congenital deformity. Fifty

Plate 40.
The Heart

HEART SEEN FROM ABOVE

Innominate and l. common carotid aa.

To entire body

L. subclav. a. and v.

L. jugular v.

R. innominate v.

L. innominate v.

Ligamentum arteriosum

Sup. vena cava

Pericardium

Phrenic n.

L. coronary ostium

Pulm. a. To lung

Pulmonary a.

Aorta

L. atrium

Pulm. vv. From lung

Valve leaflets and sinuses of Valsalva

S-A node

Fossa ovale

Mitral valve

A-V node

Ant. leaflet

Diaph.

Post. leaflet

R. atrium

Papillary mus.

Interatrial septum

L. ventricle

Orifice of coronary sinus

Interventricular septum

Inf. vena cava

Tricuspid valve

Post. leaflet

Ant. leaflet

Septal leaflet

R. ventricle

R. ventricle

R. atrium

Sup. vena cava

Inf. vena cava

Line of section

Pulmonary valve

Aortic valve

L. ant. desc. coronary a.

Circumflex a.

L. coronary ostium

Nodulus semilunaris

R. coronary ostium

Interatrial septum

Tricuspid valve

R. coronary a.

Aorta

L. coronary a.

Circumflex a.

Sinus node a.

Great cardiac v.

Vieussens' ring

Ant. cardiac vv.

L. ant. desc. coronary a.

Artery to A-V node

R. marginal a.

Interventricular septal branches

R. ventricle

L. ventricle

Post. desc. coronary a.

Ant. interventricular v.

Terminal l. ant. desc. coronary

V. of Marshall

Aorta

L. atrium

Sup. vena cava

Pulm. vv.

Coronary sinus

Inf. vena cava

L.V.

R. coronary a.

R.V.

Post. descending coronary a.

Posterior

Plate 41.
Anatomy and Physiology of the Heart

Motor and premotor areas of brain are higher centers which influence autonomic control of heart and blood pressure.

Emotional disturbances stimulate sympathetic n.

Hypothalamus translates stimuli into physiological activity.

Cardiovascular regulatory center (medulla oblongata)

Medulla

VAGUS (parasympathetic) Cardioinhibitor

SYMPATHETIC Cardioaccelerator

Ext. carotid a.

Carotid body

Branch of glossopharyngeal n.

Carotid sinus (Int. carotid a.)

R. and l. sympathetic nn.

Depression influence
Carotid sinus and aortic arch sensitive to **elevated** blood pressure and increased heart rate.

Common carotid a.

Chemoreceptors

Regulation of cardiac output and blood pressure

Pressor influence
Carotid sinus and aortic arch sensitive to **lowered** blood pressure and decreased heart rate.

Pain pathways from heart
Middle and inf. cardiac and T1–5 sympath. nn.

Aortic body

Cardiac plexus of parasympathetic (vagal) and sympathetic nn.

Pulm. a.

Aorta

L. atrium

Heartbeat
Stimuli at sinoatrial node (pacemaker) spread to atria and ventricles via atrioventricular node, thus maintaining automatic rhythm.

Sinoatrial node

R. and l. coronary aa.

Atrioventricular node

Purkinje fibers

R. atrium

L. ventricle

Bundle of His

R. ventricle

I.V.C.

Interventricular septum

R. bundle of His

L. bundle of His

thousand children are born every year with congenital malformations of the heart that include holes or defects in the atrial and ventricular septum and deformity of any of the four valves. In addition to these congenital defects, there are acquired diseases of the valves secondary to rheumatic heart disease, and, also, occlusion of the coronary arteries can result from arteriosclerosis. Most of these congenital and acquired defects can be surgically corrected, at the present time, with relatively low risk.

NEUROLOGICAL CONTROL OF HEART RATE

In the mammalian heart, there is a system of specialized tissue (junctional tissue) that possesses the property of rhythmical impulse formation and conductivity to a higher degree than the cardiac muscle itself. One tiny island of junctional tissue called the *sinoatrial node* (S-A node) has this ability to generate a rhythmical electrical impulse, and it is commonly referred to as the "pacemaker" of the heart. The S-A node is located at the junction of the superior vena cava and the right atrium, and the impulse generated by this junctional tissue spreads as an electrical wave in all directions through the muscle of the atrium. This impulse is then picked up by a second node called the *atrioventricular node* (A-V node), which is located at the base of the right atrium just above the tricuspid valve. The electrical impulse then passes from the A-V node down into the A-V bundle, and into right and left branches to all portions of both ventricles through terminal Purkinje fibers. It is this excitation wave that provides the changes in electrical potential that can be recorded as the electrocardiogram.

Although the heart has a complex neuro-control system to maintain proper heart rate and cardiac output, the totally denervated heart can respond surprisingly well to changes in its load. As demonstrated in patients with heart transplants, this is achieved primarily by the effect of catecholamine release from the adrenal medulla, as well as a second important mechanism, described many years ago by the physiologist Starling. He pointed out that if the ventricles receive an increased volume of blood, they can respond by contracting more forcibly. This obviously is an important self-regulatory mechanism for the denervated heart.

In the normal innervated heart, the primary center for control of cardiac rate is the cardiovascular regulatory center located in the medulla oblongata. This center is under constant stimulation from higher centers in the brain, centers that are primarily located in the frontal lobes, where the emotional disturbances of anger, fear, and excitement are rapidly transmitted, through the hypothalamus, as an excitatory

stimulus to the cardiovascular regulatory center.

The primary control of heart rate is through the vagus nerves arising in the region of the cardiovascular regulatory center. Stimulation of the vagus nerves causes an inhibitory effect with slowing of the heart rate and lowering of the blood pressure. The final vagal pathway to the heart is through the cardiac plexus, which is located at the bifurcation of the trachea. In addition to the vagal innervation (parasympathetic) of the heart, there is sympathetic innervation, which likewise arises from the cardiovascular regulatory center. These sympathetic fibers emerge from the cervical and upper thoracic ganglia of the sympathetic cord and pass by way of the superior, middle, and inferior cardiac nerves, again through the cardiac plexus, to the heart. Stimulation of the sympathetic fibers accelerates heart rate and increases the force of contraction.

There are some important afferent nervous reflexes that play a critical role in the rate of heart contraction. Afferent nerves arising in the right atrium can sense an increase in atrial pressure and stimulate the cardiovascular regulatory center to increase the heart rate (Bainbridge reflex). Similarly, there are afferent fibers, termed *pressoreceptors,* in the arch of the aorta and in the bifurcation of the carotid arteries, which sense an increased pressure in these vessels and in turn signal the cardiovascular regulatory center to slow down the heart rate (Marey's reflex). The afferent fibers from the pressoreceptors in the arch of the aorta and the carotid sinus pass via the vagus nerves (X) and glossopharyngeal nerves (IX) respectively, to the cardiovascular regulatory center. In addition, there are chemoreceptors located in the arterial wall at the carotid bifurcation and aortic arch that sense changes in blood pO_2, pCO_2, and pH. The afferent impulses arising in these fibers mainly alter respiration, but to a lesser degree modify heart rate and vasomotor tone. Decreasing pO_2 and pH and increasing pCO_2 not only increase the respiratory rate but accelerate the heart rate and enhance vasoconstriction. The afferent impulses from the chemoreceptors pass, with the afferent fibers, from pressoreceptors via the ninth and tenth nerves to the cardiovascular regulatory center.

An additional important set of afferent fibers are the pain fibers, which are stimulated by conditions of myocardial ischemia and cause the clinical condition of angina pectoris, or pain in the chest. These sensory fibers pass with the sympathetic nerves in the middle and inferior cardiac nerves and enter the spinal cord via the posterior roots of the upper five thoracic segments. This routing of afferent pain fibers of the heart through these upper five thoracic segments explains why the pain of myocardial ischemia is referred to the shoulders, upper extremities, and regions of the neck.

17

The Lungs

Henry N. Wagner, Jr., M.D.

In the thirteenth century ibn-an-Nafis challenged the concept of Galen that blood passes from the right side of the heart to the left via invisible pores in the cardiac septum, where it mixes with the air from the lungs to produce the vital spirit. He proposed that "in the wisdom of God," blood was carried to the lungs via the pulmonary artery so that "what seeps through the pores in the branches of this vessel into the alveoli of the lungs mixes with air and is then carried to the left chamber of the heart by the pulmonary veins." Five hundred years later, Stephen Hales elucidated the details of the relationship of structure and function in the lung. He correctly measured the dimensions of alveoli as 1/100 of an inch (254 micra) with a total surface area of about 289 square feet (27 square meters). He confirmed that this enormous surface was the site of entry of the "air particles" found in the blood and concluded that the most crucial function of the lungs is the exchange of carbon dioxide for oxygen.

Other important functions of the lung are related to the central position of the pulmonary circulation between the two chambers of the heart, and through which the entire cardiac output passes. These include sieving of particulate matter and the production and elimination of substances such as hormones from the blood.

The right lung is usually larger than the left, because of the space occupied by the heart. The left lung consists of two lobes, the right lung of three. The interlobar fissure of the left lung runs diagonally downward from a point about 6 cm from the apex of the lung to the base of the lung. The upper lobe consists of four segments: the apical-posterior, anterior, superior, and inferior lingular segments. The left lower lobe consists of a superior, anterior-medial basal, lateral basal, and posterior basal segment. The right upper lobe consists of an apical, posterior, and anterior segment; the middle lobe of a lateral and medial segment; and the lower lobe of a superior, anterior, medial, lateral, and posterior basal segment.

The airways, bronchial and pulmonary circulations, lymphatic system, and the nerves supplying the lungs make up the important structural elements of the lungs. In the adult, the pulmonary arteries accompany the airways quite closely, while pulmonary veins lie between two airway trees. Bronchovascular units consist of lobes, segments, lobules, acini, and alveoli. It has also been found useful to divide the lungs into three concentric zones. The respiratory zone consists of the alveoli, with the alveolar capillary network that consists of a waffle-like array of vessels with numerous connections. Here the alveoli and vessels are in intimate contact, which permits effective exchange of gases to take place. In the conductive zone are the bronchi, bronchioles, pulmonary arteries, and veins. Their walls separate air from blood, and regulatory mechanisms control the relative distributions of both, continually matching ventilation and perfusion in the healthy state. The transitory zone connects the other two and contains the respiratory bronchioles, alveolar ducts, and sacs, and the pre- and post-capillaries.

Electron microscopy has permitted measurement of the thickness of the alveolo-capillary tissue separating air from blood. In its thinnest portions it was found to be about 0.4 micra. In reaching this point, molecular gases traverse the airway system that distributes the air among the alveoli. During gaseous exchange, the tissues traversed by the respiratory gases comprise the alveolar epithelium, its basement membrane, a narrow connective tissue space,

Plate 42.
The Lungs, Bronchi, Pleurae, and Blood Vessels

Lower border of lung

Lower border of pleura

Cardiac notch

Ant.-post. view

L. lat. view

Thyroid cart.

Trachea

R. and l. bronchi and pulm. aa.

B1
B2
B3
B4
B5
B8
B10
B9
B6
B7
B10
B2
B1
B3
B4
B5
B8
B7

ANATOMY AND PHYSIOLOGY OF THE BRONCHIOLE

Cartilage

Bronchiole

Bronchial a.

R. and l. sup. pulm. vv.

Upper lobe lung

Upper lobe

Middle lobe

Lower lobe

R. and l. inf. pulm. vv.

Lower lobe

Lingula

Vagus n. (parasympathetic)

Sensory from mucosa and muscle

Gland and duct opening into lumen

Smooth muscle

Terminal bronchioles

Motor n. to muscle and glands. Central and reflex neural impulses produce bronchoconstriction and secretion. High-level brain impulses may produce hypersecretion and bronchoconstriction.

Sympathetic n. impulses produce bronchodilatation and vasoconstriction.

Pulmonary venule

Site of exchange of gases, oxygen, and carbon dioxide

Pulmonary a.

Alveolus

**PRIMARY LOBULE—
THE TERMINAL END OF A
BRONCHIOLE**

Respiratory bronchioles

Alveolar ducts

Atrium

Alveolar sac

Plate 43.
Lobes of the Lungs

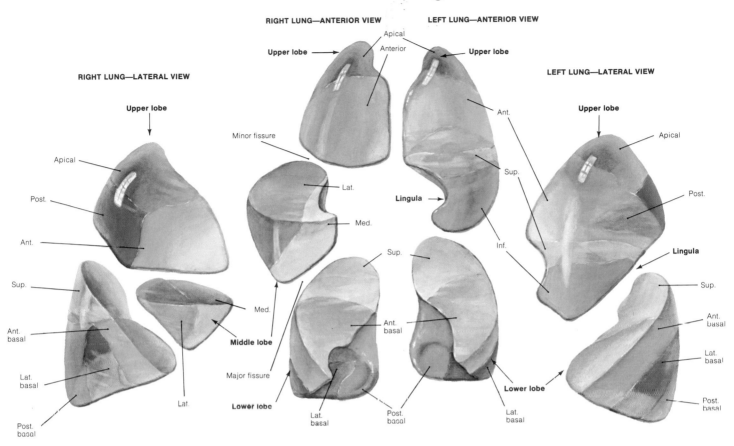

RIGHT LUNG—ANTERIOR VIEW

Apical

Anterior

Upper lobe

LEFT LUNG—ANTERIOR VIEW

Upper lobe

RIGHT LUNG—LATERAL VIEW

Upper lobe

Apical

Post.

Ant.

Sup.

Ant. basal

Lat. basal

Post. basal

Minor fissure

Lat.

Med.

Med.

Middle lobe

Major fissure

Lower lobe

Lat. basal

Post. basal

Sup.

Ant. basal

Lingula

Inf.

Ant.

Lower lobe

Lat. basal

LEFT LUNG—LATERAL VIEW

Upper lobe

Apical

Post.

Lingula

Sup.

Ant. basal

Lat. basal

Post. basal

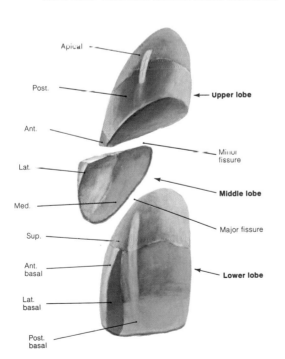

RIGHT LUNG—POSTERIOR ASPECTS VIEWED ANTERIORLY

Apical

Post.

Ant.

Lat.

Med.

Sup.

Ant. basal

Lat. basal

Post. basal

Upper lobe

Minor fissure

Middle lobe

Major fissure

Lower lobe

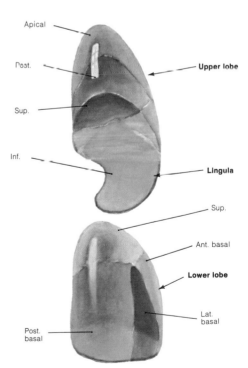

LEFT LUNG—POSTERIOR ASPECTS VIEWED ANTERIORLY

Apical

Post.

Sup.

Inf.

Upper lobe

Lingula

Sup.

Ant. basal

Lower lobe

Lat. basal

Post. basal

the basement membrane of the capillary endothelium, and the capillary endothelium itself. Because of the low pressure in the lungs, the slightest variation in resistance to blood flow either in the vessels themselves or transmitted to the vessels from the alveoli has a great effect on local pulmonary blood flow. The distribution of the pulmonary circulation is therefore in a continual state of change as the result of postural changes, exercise, and other factors. With work or other exercise, the exchange of respiratory gases is increased by more active pulmonary ventilation and an increase in pulmonary arterial blood flow. For this gaseous exchange to be efficient, changes in regional blood flow must match the changes in ventilation. In most diseases, whenever regional ventilation is impaired the pulmonary arterial blood flow to the involved zones decreases as the result of arteriolar constriction. In some diseases, however, the disease is at a level where perfusion and ventilation are no longer matched and cyanosis results. In other diseases, perfusion is reduced without impairment of ventilation. Of these, pulmonary embolism is the most common. In most patients, such emboli are larger than the 2-mm diameter of the segmental pulmonary arteries, and perfusion defects corresponding to specific lung segments can be seen. Diagnostic specificity can be increased if attention is paid to the size, shape, and location of perfusion defects, as seen in lung scans or pulmonary arteriograms.

Although dyspnea with exercise is the most common and perhaps the most sensitive indicator of lung disease, measurement of properties of the lungs such as size, volume of the air spaces, expansibility (compliance or airway resistance), ventilatory ability (vital capacity, maximal breathing capacity) and rate of gas exchange (diffusing capacity), together with regional measurements of ventilation and perfusion, give us a more detailed picture of the gas-exchange function of the lungs. In many cases identification of the pattern of abnormalities can help elucidate the probable cause of the disease in a given patient, help predict what is likely to happen to him, and provide the basis for more rational treatment.

Other functions of the lung are also of great importance: these include coughing, mucociliary activity, and alveolar phagocytosis. These can be examined with a variety of techniques, many of them involving direct measurements with radioactive tracers. These help in two ways: (1) to define abnormalities of individual lung functions in precise quantitative terms; and (2) to locate the areas of function in terms of segments and lobes at the gross anatomic level, or at the microscopic level, at the alveolar, interstitial, bronchial or vascular levels. Such information is useful in planning treatment and in objective evaluation of the results of treatment.

18

The Gastrointestinal Tract

Thomas R. Hendrix, M.D.
George D. Zuidema, M.D.
John J. White, M.D.

EMBRYOLOGY

A knowledge of the embryological development of the abdominal viscera is basic to an understanding of the normal relationships that these viscera assume as well as necessary for explaining the congenital malformations that are encountered with reasonable frequency. The embryonic gut is a simple tubular structure that lies suspended from the ventral and dorsal walls of the developing embryo by double-layered ventral and dorsal mesenteries. Fairly early in embryological development the caudal portion of the ventral mesentery disappears, and there is free communication between the right and left portions of the abdominal cavity. The cranial portion of the ventral mesentery persists, however, and is the site for the development of the liver. The portion of ventral mesentery lying between the liver and the ventral abdominal wall persists as the falciform ligament. The lower free margin of this ligament contains the obliterated left umbilical vein, the ligamentum teres. The persistent portion of ventral mesentery between the liver and stomach becomes the gastrohepatic ligament, or lesser omentum. This extends to the duodenum and at its lower margin contains the common bile duct, hepatic artery, and portal vein.

The portion of the original dorsal mesentery that suspends the stomach is termed the mesogastrium; that part suspending the jejunum and ileum is termed dorsal mesentry; and the portion supporting the colon is the mesocolon. The spleen develops in the cranial portion of the dorsal mesentery and the vascular supply to the foregut arises partially from the celiac axis. The branches of the celiac axis lie between the layers of dorsal mesentery. The hepatic artery supplies the liver, the left gastric artery supplies the stomach, and the splenic artery supplies the spleen. The persistent dorsal mesentery between stomach and spleen is termed the gastrosplenic ligament, and the mesenteric attachment between the spleen and the midline is the splenoaortic ligament.

The foregut undergoes a 90-degree rotation to the right about the longitudinal axis of the stomach. As a result of this rotation the dorsal border of the stomach, the greater omentum, and the spleen become located in the left upper quadrant. A remnant of the splenoaortic ligament becomes the splenorenal ligament.

The foregut undergoes a second phase of rotation in relation to the horizontal axis of the stomach as a result of the unequal rates of growth of the rapidly expanding dorsal mesentery and the slowly growing ventral mesentery. The ventral mesentery fixes the location of the lesser curvature of the stomach while the greater curvature continues to expand. This brings the pyloric end of the stomach upward and to the right where it becomes fixed in position. The dorsal mesogastrium, by its displacement, creates a large sac posterior to the stomach termed the *omental bursa*. The dorsal mesentery is now named greater omentum. A small opening between the greater peritoneal cavity and the omental bursa persists as the foramen of Winslow. The boundaries of this opening include the caudate lobe of the liver above; the duodenum below; the hepatoduodenal ligament containing hepatic artery, common bile duct, and portal vein in front; and the inferior vena cava behind.

The greater omentum is formed by the fusion of the anterior and posterior layers of the original dorsal mesentery. The area that persists posterior to the transverse colon constitutes the transverse mesocolon; the anterior layers constitute the gastrocolic ligament.

Plate 44.
Intestinal Rotation (Fetus)

Greater omentum

Aorta

Parietal peritoneum

Celiac a.

Foregut

Sup. mesenteric a.

Liver

Rotation to the right

Inf. mesenteric a.

Umbilical cord

Rotation to the left

Cecum

Omphalomesenteric vess. and obliterated duct

Rotation of midgut within exocoelomic cavity

Hindgut

Compression of duodenum by sup. mesenteric a.

Aorta

Pancreas

Fat pad

Distended proximal duodenum

Normal

SUPERIOR MESENTERY ARTERY SYNDROME

Rotation of the Midgut

During embryological development the primitive tubular midgut is suspended by a dorsal mesentery which divides posteriorly over the retroperitoneal area and continues over the posterior abdominal wall as parietal peritoneum. The midgut extends from the duodenojejunal junction to midtransverse colon. Its blood supply is by the superior mesenteric artery which lies between the two layers of dorsal mesentery and extends into the yolk sac as the vitelline artery. The superior mesenteric artery serves as the axis of rotation of the midgut. Rotation occurs in three stages: the first consists of physiologic herniation into the exocoelomic cavity; in the second phase the viscera return to the developing peritoneal or coelomic cavity; the third stage consists of fixation of the viscera into their final locations. Both rotation and mobilization of the intestinal tract occur during all three stages. During the first stage the midgut undergoes rapid elongation. This growth extends to the point at which the coelomic cavity is no longer capable of accommodating it. Consequently, it herniates through the umbilical orifice into the primitive umbilical cord. The superior mesenteric artery is the major structure within the herniated loop which is attached at its other end to the yolk stalk. During this exocoelomic phase the midgut undergoes a 90-degree counterclockwise rotation which throws the cranial portion of the loop to the right and the caudal portion to the left.

As the coelomic cavity enlarges, the midgut returns, retreating from its exocoelomic location. This phase is extremely important, for a further counterclockwise rotation of 180 degrees occurs. The superior mesenteric artery remains as the axis of rotation during this phase of reduction. The proximal portion of the cranial loop is reduced first, passing under the superior mesenteric artery. The caudal loop is the last to reenter the abdominal cavity after completion of the rotation. Upon completion of this stage the cecum and proximal colon (distal portion of caudal loop) become situated in the right upper quadrant of the abdomen. This stage completes the rotation of the midgut.

During the final, or fixation, stage the cecum descends from its subhepatic location to its normal position in the right side of the peritoneal cavity. The dorsal mesentery of the cecum and ascending colon becomes obliterated and fixed to the parietal peritoneum in the right flank. The transverse colon remains suspended from the transverse mesocolon from the hepatic flexure to the splenic flexure. The mesentery of the small bowel extends from the duodenojejunal junction at the ligament of Treitz to the ileocolic valve; the mesenteric base is attached along an oblique line extending downward from the ligament of Treitz toward the right lower quadrant. On the left side the descending colon loses its peritoneum and becomes fused along the left lateral posterior peritoneal wall, and only the sigmoid colon retains a mesentery.

A variety of congenital malformations of the abdominal viscera may result from abnormal patterns of rotation, particularly involving the midgut. The anatomical relationships of the umbilical region of the fetus at term are also shown. At this stage the ductus arteriosus is patent, as are the sinus venosus and umbilical vein, the urachus and the hypogastric arteries. The umbilical veins and the hypogastric arteries are combined as the omphalomesenteric vessels within the umbilicus. These structures become obliterated as does the sinus venosus as the fetus begins extra-uterine life. Failure of these structures to obliterate leads to a variety of congenital malformations, samples of which are described. An omphalocele (not shown) results when rotation fails to continue beyond the first stage and the midgut remains arrested within exocoelomic cavity. The loop of bowel is covered by amnion and the abdominal wall may be incompletely developed so that a massive defect may be present. The hernia may consist of a single loop of bowel or may contain virtually the entire intestinal tract, liver, spleen, and pancreas.

Several important anomalies may be produced by irregularities of rotation and fixation of the midgut. Failure of the stage of fixation (stage three) may result in the cecum occupying a subhepatic location. If the visceral peritoneum fails to fuse with the posterior parietal peritoneum, the entire cecum and ascending colon remain free on a mesentery and mobile. This makes cecal volvulus possible.

The most common anomaly of intestinal rotation is encountered when the appendix becomes fixed under the cecum during its descent into the right lower quadrant. The appendix then persists in a retroperitoneal or retrocecal location (not shown).

In the early human embryo the umbilical loop of the primitive gut communicates freely with the yolk sac by way of the omphalomesenteric duct. As development proceeds, this duct normally becomes occluded and later disappears entirely. All or any part of the duct may, however, persist. If the duct remains attenuated, but with an intact lumen, an umbilico-intestinal fistula results. The remnant of the duct may be very short so that the ileum appears to be attached to the undersurface of the abdominal wall, or it may be several inches in length. A variety of anomalous arrangements may result, ranging from an open communication with prolapse of the bowel through the opening, producing intestinal obstruction, to a very narrow lumen which is productive of only a small mucous discharge.

If the midportion of the duct remains present, an

Plate 45.
Small Intestinal Malformations—
Embryological Considerations

Umbilical region of fetus at term (after Max Brödel)

Patent ductus

Aorta

Ductus venosus

Sup. mesenteric a.

Portal v.

Umbilical v.

Umbilicus

Omphalomesenteric vess.

Allantois

Urachus

Hypogastric aa.

Bladder

Ileum

Umbilicus

Omphalomesenteric vess.

**PERSISTENT OMPHALOMESENTERIC DUCT
(MECKEL'S DIVERTICULUM)**

**PERSISTENT OMPHALOMESENTERIC DUCT
UMBILICO-INTESTINAL FISTULA**

Ileum

INTESTINAL CYST

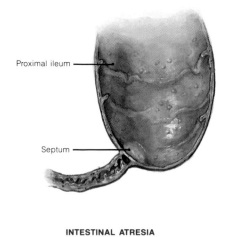

Proximal ileum

Septum

INTESTINAL ATRESIA

intestinal cyst may occur. This cyst may communicate with the umbilicus or the ileum, or only the middle portion may persist as a blind cyst.

If the proximal portion of the omphalomesenteric duct remains persistent, a blind diverticulum attached to the ileum results. This is termed Meckel's diverticulum and is a very common anomaly of the intestinal tract. It is usually located within a meter of the terminal ileum and may or may not have an associated mesentery.

In addition to anomalies in the rotational and fixation phases of midgut development, anomalies may also be encountered as a result of failure of lumen development, such as atresia, stenosis, or duplication of the bowel lumen. During the sixth week of embryonic life the epithelial lining of the gut proliferates rapidly. This results in temporary obliteration of the lumen to varying degrees. Later, vacuoles appear within the solid epithelial cord of the alimentary tract. As the vacuoles coalesce, normal lumen patency occurs. Failure of coalescence of the vacuoles, however, may result in persistence of a transverse septum and obliteration of the lumen, resulting in intestinal atresia. Stenosis may be the result of a variant in this same process in which the transverse septum undergoes incomplete resolution.

An alternate theory to explain the development of intestinal atresia or stenosis is based on the hypothesis that local abnormalities in the blood supply occur, producing small areas of vascular insufficiency, leading to abnormalities in development. An intestinal duplication, with development of an enteric or enterogenous cyst, results when the vacuolation produces a longitudinal septum. Duplication cysts may occur in any portion of the alimentary tract, and they usually do not communicate with the intestinal lumen.

The urachus is a midline fibrous cord extending from the apex of the bladder to the umbilicus. During embryonic life, this structure is the allantoic stalk. If the lumen is persistent, the result is a fistula between the umbilicus and the urinary bladder.

Another variation that may be encountered is a state in which the intestinal tract returns to the coelomic cavity but rotation beyond the initial 90-degree turn is arrested. This results in placing the cranial limb of the embryonic midgut in the right side of the peritoneal cavity and the caudal limb in the left side so that in the fetus the small intestine lies entirely on the right side of the abdomen, with the cecum and the entire large bowel located on the left. This anomaly may be completely asymptomatic and detected only when barium studies are performed for some other reason later in life. It may be particularly troublesome if appendicitis develops in a patient with this aberrant condition.

In rare instances reversed rotation (clockwise) may occur during the stage of reduction into the coelomic cavity. In this situation the duodenum lies anterior to the superior mesenteric artery and the transverse colon arises behind. As the root of mesentery becomes fixed, the transverse colon may be obstructed by the superior mesenteric artery.

If intestinal rotation is arrested upon the completion of stage two, fixation of the mesentery fails to occur, and the entire midgut loop hangs from a narrow pedicle based on the superior mesenteric vessels. This arrangement predisposes to volvulus of the bowel around the superior mesenteric vessels. In the worst situation this may result in extensive intestinal infarction. More often the patient may present with symptoms of partial or complete duodenal obstruction dating from birth.

Internal hernias may result if the returning cranial loop of midgut rotates into the mesentery of the caudal loop rather than into the general peritoneal cavity. With fixation of the mesentery loop the bowel may become imprisoned beneath the mesentery, and a paraduodenal hernia may result.

ANATOMY

The mouth and pharynx serve as the entrance to both the respiratory and gastrointestinal tracts. The oropharyngeal musculature is striated and is innervated by the cranial nerves. Its complex, stereotyped activities are coordinated by centers in the brain stem (medulla oblongata), e.g., the swallowing center, respiratory center, vomiting center, etc. The mouth and pharynx are lined with stratified squamous epithelium and lubricated by the secretion of the simple buccal glands and the complex salivary glands, the parotid, submaxillary, and sublingual glands.

The esophagus is the conduit connecting the pharynx to the stomach. Its muscular coat is composed of two layers, an outer one with longitudinally arranged fibers and an inner one with circularly arranged fibers. The upper one-third of the esophageal musculature is striated muscle, whereas the lower two-thirds are smooth. The extrinsic innervation of the esophagus is from the esophageal plexus. The esophagus is also lined with stratified squamous epithelium. It passes down the posterior mediastinum through the esophageal hiatus in the diaphragm, to enter the stomach in the abdomen.

The arterial blood supply of the esophagus is segmental in nature, with the upper portion derived from the inferior thyroid artery, the midportion arising from esophageal branches of the intercostal and bronchial arteries, and the lowermost part supplied by ascending branches of the left gastric artery. The venous drainage is via the azygos vein into the supe-

Plate 46.
Esophagus—Arteries and Nerves

Thyroid cart.

Cricoid cart.

Trachea

Thyroid

Esophagus

Recurrent laryngeal n.

Splanchnic n. (sympathetic)

Esophageal branch from left gastric a.

Aortic hiatus (medial arcuate lig.)

Right crus diaphragm

Azygos v. and splanchnic n.

Sympathetic trunk

Lumbar lymphatic trunks

Third lumbar vertebra

Vagus n. (parasympathetic)

Sympathetic n. trunk

Thyropharyngeal mus.

Cricopharyngeal mus.

Inf. thyroid a.

Thyrocervical trunk

Left subclavian a.

Esophageal branch

Aorta

Esophageal branch from bronchial a.

Heart

Esophageal branch from intercostal a.

Esophageal branch from left inf. phrenic a.

Ant. and post. vagus nn.

Inf. phrenic a.

Celiac lymph nodes

Thoracic duct

Intestinal lymphatic trunk

Left crus diaphragm

Cisterna chyli

rior vena cava above, and by the coronary vein, entering the portal vein below.

The stomach is fixed at its two poles, the esophagogastric junction and the gastroduodenal junction. The proximal stomach, or fundus, lies high in the left upper quadrant of the abdomen under the diaphragm. The body of the stomach courses anteriorly and to the right, where it becomes the gastric antrum, which crosses the spine anterior to the pancreas to join the duodenum, which is located retroperitoneally. The stomach has three coats of smooth muscle: an outer longitudinal, a middle circular, and an inner oblique coat. The stomach is lined by two types of glandular mucosa, which are arranged in folds, or rugae. The proximal two-thirds is the fundic mucosa, with glands containing the acid-producing parietal cells and the pepsin-producing chief cells. Antral mucosa lining the distal one-third has glands containing mucin-producing cells and G, or gastrin-producing, cells. The surface of both types of mucosa is covered by mucus-secreting cells.

Extrinsic stimulation of gastric secretion and motility arrive via the vagus nerves, which enter the abdomen along with the esophagus. Vagotomy, the interruption of vagal impulses to the parietal cell gland area and the antrum, is often used in combination with a gastric drainage procedure in the treatment of patients with duodenal ulcer. In a truncal vagotomy, the primary vagal trunks are sectioned. In a selective vagotomy, the major branches to the stomach are cut but the hepatic branches are preserved. In parietal cell vagotomy, or highly selective vagotomy, the hepatic and antral branches are preserved, and only those branches to the fundus and body of the stomach are cut.

The arterial blood supply of the stomach comes from the celiac axis. The left gastric artery supplies the lower esophagus and the lesser curvature of the fundus and body of the stomach. The hepatic artery branch of the celiac axis gives rise to the right gastric artery to the antrum and the gastroduodenum and continues along the greater curvature as the right gastroepiploic artery. The splenic artery gives off the left gastroepiploic artery, which furnishes the blood supply to the greater curvature aspect of the body and fundus. The collateral circulation of the stomach is extensive, and it is usually possible to ligate two of the main arteries without devascularizing the stomach. The venous drainage parallels the arterial supply and enters the portal system. These collateral veins are of clinical importance in the presence of portal hypertension.

The primary venous drainage of the stomach and intestines is the portal vein, formed by the confluence of the superior mesenteric and splenic veins. The inferior mesenteric vein enters the splenic vein a short distance from the origin of the portal vein, and

the coronary vein draining the stomach also enters close to the confluence of superior mesenteric and splenic veins. When portal vein obstruction occurs, collaterals develop to the systemic venous circulation through a variety of pathways. The coronary vein connects through submucosal vessels in the esophagus and, hence, from esophageal veins to the azygous system. Increased pressure and flow through this channel causes esophageal varices. The umbilical vein may recanalize and drain to abdominal wall vessels. There are extensive collaterals in the pelvis through the hemorrhoidal system. Collaterals may develop from the base of the mesentery into retroperitoneal veins and, hence, into the lumbar veins. The hepatic veins are very short and enter directly into the vena cava just before it enters the right atrium.

The duodenum, the first portion of the small intestine, is retroperitoneal. It curves around the head of the pancreas, crosses the spine along the lower margin of the pancreas, and reenters the peritoneal cavity at the ligament of Treitz, where it becomes the jejunum. The duodenum receives the acid gastric chyme and the alkaline secretions of the pancreas and liver, as well as the secretion of the many mucosal Brunner's glands. The small intestine, duodenum, jejunum, and ileum all have two muscular coats, an outer longitudinal and inner circular coat. The small intestine is lined with columnal epithelium arranged in tall finger- and leaflike projections, or villi, and short tibular glands, the crypts of Lieberkühn. In addition the mucosa is arranged in circular folds called *valvulae conniventes*. The jejunum and ileum are suspended in the abdomen on the mesentery, which contains the arteries, veins, lymphatics, and nerves serving the intestine. The superior mesenteric artery provides the major blood supply to the jejunum and ileum.

In the right lower quadrant of the abdomen, the ileum enters the medial side of the cecum, the proximal portion of the colon. The appendix, a vestigial structure in man, is located at the dependent, blind end of the cecum. The ascending colon passes from the cecum in the right lower quadrant up to the hepatic flexure under the liver in the right upper quadrant. From this point, the transverse colon crosses to the left upper quadrant, where at the splenic flexure it becomes the descending colon.

As the colon enters the left lower quadrant of the abdomen, it becomes the sigmoid colon. It leaves the peritoneal cavity posterior to the bladder to become the rectum, and opens onto the perineum through the anal canal.

The colonic wall consists of mucosa, submucosa, a circular layer of smooth muscle, a longitudinal layer of smooth muscle and a serosal lining. The external surface of the colon has three characteristic struc-

Plate 47.
The Stomach—Neural Considerations

Hypothalamus

Normal and disturbed physiology (e.g., psychic) reflected via vagus (parasympathetic) and splanchnic (sympathetic) nerves

Secretions and motility of stomach regulated by autonomic nervous system

Vagus nerve

Esophagus

Splanchnic nerve

Celiac ganglion and plexus

Duodenum

Fundus

Cardia

Body

Transitional

Antral

Parasympathetic stimulation— vagus nerve
Increased secretory activity, tone, and peristalsis

Sympathetic stimulation— splanchnic nerve
Decreased secretory activity, tone, and peristalsis

Fundal zone— acid and pepsin secretion (gastric juice)

Antral zone— alkaline mucus secretion. Secretes hormone gastrin into bloodstream.

Surface epithelium

Gastric pits

Visceral afferent pathway

Gastric glands

Secretion and peristalsis also controlled locally by intrinsic mixed sympathetic nerves—myenteric and submucosal plexuses

Muscularis mucosa

Pathologic response— gastric juice, rich in HCl and pepsin, may penetrate protective mucus coating, rendering mucosa vulnerable to erosion and ulceration.

Submucosa

Smooth muscle

Serosa

BLOCK OF STOMACH WALL

Plate 48.
Pancreas and Stomach

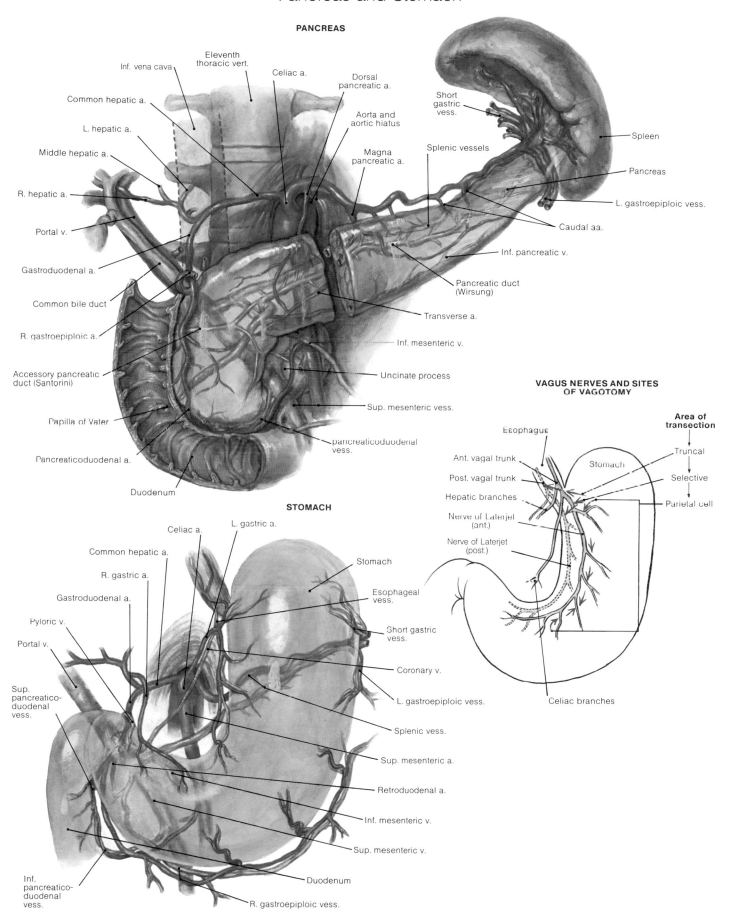

PANCREAS

Inf. vena cava

Eleventh thoracic vert.

Celiac a.

Common hepatic a.

Dorsal pancreatic a.

Aorta and aortic hiatus

L. hepatic a.

Magna pancreatic a.

Short gastric vess.

Splenic vessels

Spleen

Middle hepatic a.

Pancreas

R. hepatic a.

L. gastroepiploic vess.

Portal v.

Caudal aa.

Gastroduodenal a.

Inf. pancreatic v.

Common bile duct

Pancreatic duct (Wirsung)

R. gastroepiploic a.

Transverse a.

Accessory pancreatic duct (Santorini)

Inf. mesenteric v.

Uncinate process

Papilla of Vater

Sup. mesenteric vess.

Pancreaticoduodenal a.

pancreaticoduodenal vess.

Duodenum

STOMACH

Celiac a.

L. gastric a.

Stomach

Common hepatic a.

Esophageal vess.

R. gastric a.

Short gastric vess.

Gastroduodenal a.

Pyloric v.

Coronary v.

Portal v.

L. gastroepiploic vess.

Splenic vess.

Sup. pancreatico-duodenal vess.

Sup. mesenteric a.

Retroduodenal a.

Inf. mesenteric v.

Sup. mesenteric v.

Inf. pancreatico-duodenal vess.

Duodenum

R. gastroepiploic vess.

VAGUS NERVES AND SITES OF VAGOTOMY

Esophagus

Area of transection

Ant. vagal trunk

Stomach

Truncal

Post. vagal trunk

Selective

Hepatic branches

Parietal cell

Nerve of Laterjet (ant.)

Nerve of Laterjet (post.)

Celiac branches

Plate 49.
Esophagus—Liver
Venous Drainage and Collateral Channels

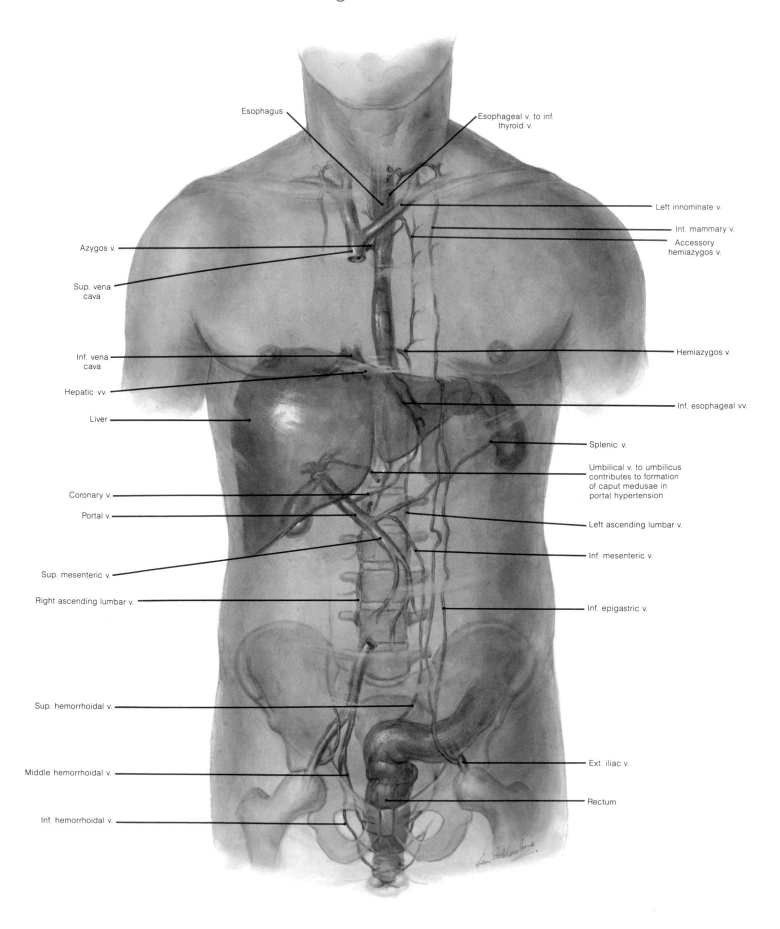

Esophagus

Esophageal v. to inf. thyroid v.

Left innominate v.

Int. mammary v.

Accessory hemiazygos v.

Azygos v.

Sup. vena cava

Inf. vena cava

Hepatic vv.

Liver

Coronary v.

Portal v.

Sup. mesenteric v.

Right ascending lumbar v.

Sup. hemorrhoidal v.

Middle hemorrhoidal v.

Inf. hemorrhoidal v.

Hemiazygos v.

Inf. esophageal vv.

Splenic v.

Umbilical v. to umbilicus contributes to formation of caput medusae in portal hypertension

Left ascending lumbar v.

Inf. mesenteric v.

Inf. epigastric v.

Ext. iliac v.

Rectum

Plate 50.
The Small Intestine

Descending portion of duodenum

Peritoneum

Kidney

Superior portion of duodenum

Pylorus

Ligament of Treitz

Duodenojejunal junction

Middle colic vess.

Inf. pancreaticoduodenal vess.

Sup. mesenteric vess.

Transverse portion of duodenum

Root mesentery small intestine

R. colic vess.

Jejunal and ileal vess.

Small intestine (jejunum)

Ileocolic vess.

Terminal ileum

Cecum

Appendix and vess.

MECHANISM OF COLONIC MOVEMENT

Water-absorbing cells

Goblet mucus-producing cells provide protective and lubricating coating.

Colon

Peristaltic contractions

Pressure, distension, and/or surface irritant produce (1) analward relaxation wave and (2) proximal peristalsis.

Relaxation wave

Analward

Crypt of Lieberkühn

Mucosa

Muscularis mucosa

Meissner plexus

Submucosa

Circular muscle

Auerbach plexus

Longitudinal muscle

Serosa

Intrinsic nerves

Extrinsic nerves

Contraction (parasympathetic)

Relaxation (sympathetic)

Plate 51.
Colon, Rectum, Anus, and Perineum

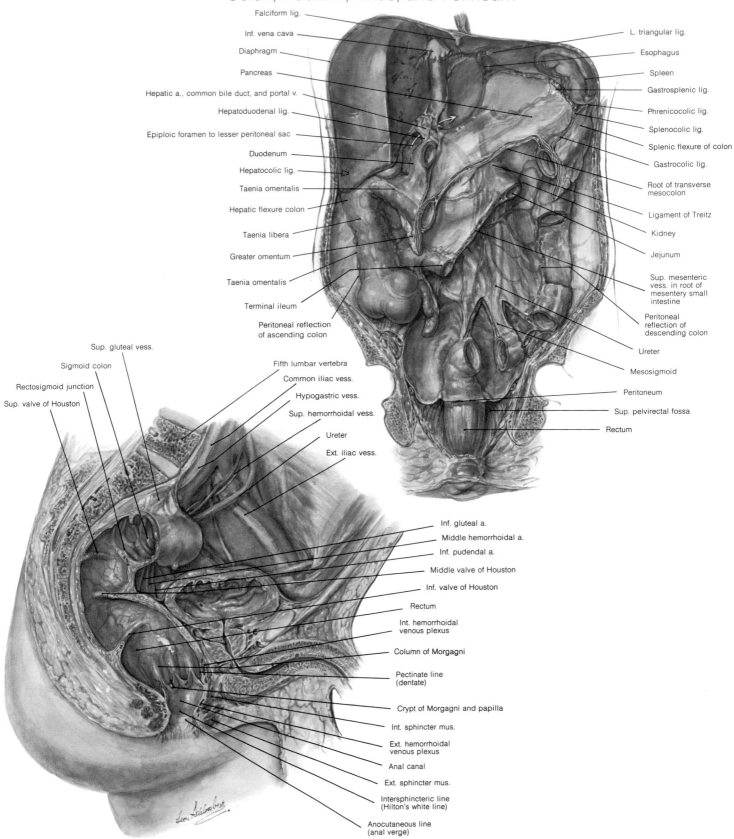

Falciform lig.

Inf. vena cava

Diaphragm

Pancreas

Hepatic a., common bile duct, and portal v.

Hepatoduodenal lig.

Epiploic foramen to lesser peritoneal sac

Duodenum

Hepatocolic lig.

Taenia omentalis

Hepatic flexure colon

Taenia libera

Greater omentum

Taenia omentalis

Terminal ileum

Peritoneal reflection of ascending colon

L. triangular lig.

Esophagus

Spleen

Gastrosplenic lig.

Phrenicocolic lig.

Splenocolic lig.

Splenic flexure of colon

Gastrocolic lig.

Root of transverse mesocolon

Ligament of Treitz

Kidney

Jejunum

Sup. mesenteric vess. in root of mesentery small intestine

Peritoneal reflection of descending colon

Ureter

Mesosigmoid

Peritoneum

Sup. pelvirectal fossa

Rectum

Sup. gluteal vess.

Sigmoid colon

Rectosigmoid junction

Sup. valve of Houston

Fifth lumbar vertebra

Common iliac vess.

Hypogastric vess.

Sup. hemorrhoidal vess.

Ureter

Ext. iliac vess.

Inf. gluteal a.

Middle hemorrhoidal a.

Inf. pudendal a.

Middle valve of Houston

Inf. valve of Houston

Rectum

Int. hemorrhoidal venous plexus

Column of Morgagni

Pectinate line (dentate)

Crypt of Morgagni and papilla

Int. sphincter mus.

Ext. hemorrhoidal venous plexus

Anal canal

Ext. sphincter mus.

Intersphincteric line (Hilton's white line)

Anocutaneous line (anal verge)

tures: (1) the taeniae coli; (2) the haustral markings; and (3) the appendices epiploicae. The three taeniae coli are longitudinal bands which run the entire length of the colon and represent thickened portions of the longitudinal muscle layer. The haustral markings are sacculations formed in the spaces between the taeniae coli and are separated from each other by the circular layer of smooth muscle. The haustral markings are most prominent when the taeniae coli are contracted. The appendices epiploicae are small sacs filled with fat which are located beneath the serosa.

The blood supply of the ascending and transverse colons is furnished by the ileocolic and middle-colic branches of the superior mesenteric artery; and the descending and sigmoid colons are supplied by the left colic and sigmoidal branches of the inferior mesenteric artery.

The ileocolic artery arises from the right side of the distal superior mesenteric artery and supplies the appendix, cecum, and terminal ileum. The cecum and the ascending colon receive their blood supply from the right colic artery, which comes off the right side of the distal superior mesenteric artery. The right colic artery has extensive anastomoses with the ileocolic and middle colic arteries via the arcades of the marginal artery. The transverse colon is supplied by the middle colic artery arising from the superior mesenteric artery. This vessel has anastomotic connections with the right colic artery and also with the inferior mesenteric artery via the arcades of the marginal artery. The left colon and sigmoid colon receive their blood supply from the inferior mesenteric artery, which arises from the distal aorta below the renal arteries. The inferior mesenteric artery branches into the left colic artery, which supplies the proximal left colon, and the sigmoid artery, which supplies the distal left colon and sigmoid colon. It terminates as the superior hemorrhoidal artery supplying the proximal rectum. The marginal artery of Drummond consists of anastomotic arcades that connect the ileocolic, the right colic, and the middle colic arteries, which arise from the superior mesenteric artery, to the left colic and sigmoid arteries, which arise from the inferior mesenteric artery.

The proximal rectum is supplied by the superior hemorrhoidal artery. It also receives branches from the middle sacral artery, which arises from the distal aorta. The midportion of the rectum is supplied by the paired middle hemorrhoidal arteries, which arise from the hypogastric, or internal iliac, arteries. The distal rectum and anal canal are supplied by the paired inferior hemorrhoidal arteries, which arise from the internal iliac arteries.

The veins of the colon accompany the arterial branches and have similar names. The ileocolic, right colic, and middle colic veins, the venous drainage of the right colon and transverse colon, drain into the superior mesenteric vein, which joins the splenic vein behind the neck of the pancreas to form the portal vein. The left colic, sigmoidal, and superior hemorrhoidal veins join to form the inferior mesenteric vein, which drains into the splenic vein. The superior hemorrhoidal plexus is located in the submucosa of the lower rectum. The vessels of this plexus form the superior hemorrhoidal veins, which drain into the portal system via the inferior mesenteric vein. Dilatations of these veins are called internal hemorrhoids.

The external hemorrhoidal plexus is located below the pectinate line in the submucosa of the anal canal and the subcutaneous tissues of the perianal area. These drain into the systemic venous system via the inferior hemorrhoidal veins and internal iliac venous systems. Dilatations of these veins are called external hemorrhoids.

Lymphatic Drainage

Collecting lymphatic channels leave the wall of the small bowel at its mesenteric border. There are three groups of regional lymph nodes: a peripheral group located near the mesenteric border adjacent to the bowel wall; a middle group located with the small bowel mesentery; and a central group of nodes which are preaortic in location adjacent to the superior mesenteric artery. The mesenteric lymph nodes comprising these three groups are very numerous and widely distributed.

The lymphatic channels drain into the cisterna chyli which is located deep to the duodenum adjacent to the vertebral body of L2. This lymphatic channel enters the thoracic cavity by passing through the aortic hiatus to become the thoracic duct.

The nerve supply of the small intestine is derived from the superior mesenteric and celiac plexuses of the sympathetic system and from the vagus nerves. The plexuses lie adjacent to the superior mesenteric artery and celiac axis, and the distribution of nerve fibers follows the general course of these vessels. The plexuses contain both sympathetic and parasympathetic fibers. Pain associated with a lesion of the small bowel is referred to areas supplied by the ninth, tenth, and eleventh thoracic nerves. In clinical presentation the pain is usually experienced in the area of the umbilicus, and only occasionally will it spread to involve the lumbar region and the back.

The pancreas is a retroperitoneal structure lying across the upper abdomen. It has both an endocrine function provided by the islets of Langerhans (insulin and glucagon being the most important products) and an exocrine function. The digestive enzymes are produced in the pancreatic acini, and the pancreatic

Plate 52.
Colon, Rectum, and Anus—Blood Vessels

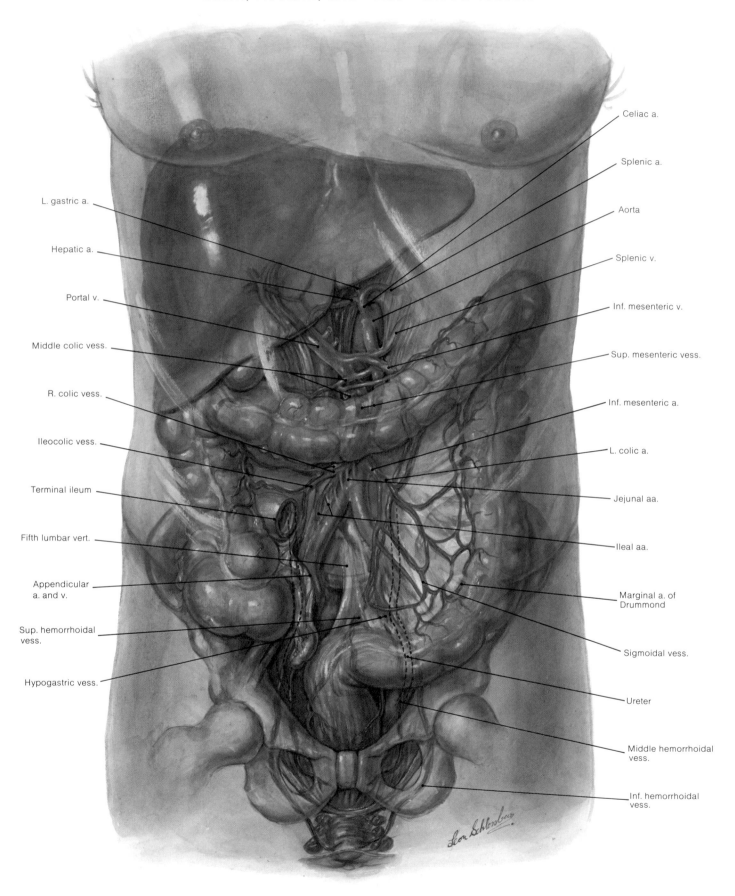

L. gastric a.

Hepatic a.

Portal v.

Middle colic vess.

R. colic vess.

Ileocolic vess.

Terminal ileum

Fifth lumbar vert.

Appendicular
a. and v.

Sup. hemorrhoidal
vess.

Hypogastric vess.

Celiac a.

Splenic a.

Aorta

Splenic v.

Inf. mesenteric v.

Sup. mesenteric vess.

Inf. mesenteric a.

L. colic a.

Jejunal aa.

Ileal aa.

Marginal a. of
Drummond

Sigmoidal vess.

Ureter

Middle hemorrhoidal
vess.

Inf. hemorrhoidal
vess.

Plate 53.
Colon, Rectum, and Anus Innervation

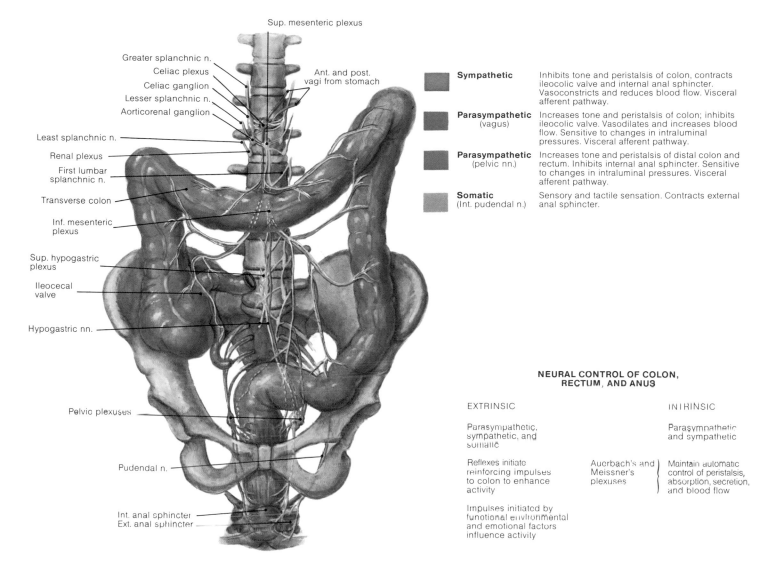

Sup. mesenteric plexus

Greater splanchnic n.
Celiac plexus
Celiac ganglion
Lesser splanchnic n.
Aorticorenal ganglion

Ant. and post. vagi from stomach

Least splanchnic n.
Renal plexus
First lumbar splanchnic n.
Transverse colon
Inf. mesenteric plexus
Sup. hypogastric plexus
Ileocecal valve
Hypogastric nn.

Pelvic plexuses

Pudendal n.

Int. anal sphincter
Ext. anal sphincter

Sympathetic	Inhibits tone and peristalsis of colon, contracts ileocolic valve and internal anal sphincter. Vasoconstricts and reduces blood flow. Visceral afferent pathway.
Parasympathetic (vagus)	Increases tone and peristalsis of colon; inhibits ileocolic valve. Vasodilates and increases blood flow. Sensitive to changes in intraluminal pressures. Visceral afferent pathway.
Parasympathetic (pelvic nn.)	Increases tone and peristalsis of distal colon and rectum. Inhibits internal anal sphincter. Sensitive to changes in intraluminal pressures. Visceral afferent pathway.
Somatic (Int. pudendal n.)	Sensory and tactile sensation. Contracts external anal sphincter.

NEURAL CONTROL OF COLON, RECTUM, AND ANUS

EXTRINSIC

Parasympathetic, sympathetic, and somatic

Reflexes initiate reinforcing impulses to colon to enhance activity

Impulses initiated by functional environmental and emotional factors influence activity

INTRINSIC

Parasympathetic and sympathetic

Auerbach's and Meissner's plexuses

Maintain automatic control of peristalsis, absorption, secretion, and blood flow

COLON (CROSS-SECTION)

Mesocolon
Marginal a.
Thickened longitudinal mus. (post. taenia)
Short branch
Long branch
Longitudinal mus.
Ant. taenia
Haustra

Lat. taenia
Semilunar fold
Thickened circular mus. attached to fixed longitudinal mus. Contraction produces clefts and haustra.

secretion is carried by the pancreatic duct to enter, with the common bile duct, the second portion of the duodenum through the ampulla of Vater.

The exocrine secretions of the pancreas enter the duodenum via the main pancreatic duct at the ampulla of Vater, or the accessory pancreatic duct (Santorini). The gastroduodenal artery lies on the head of the pancreas adjacent to the second portion of the duodenum. This vessel is essential for nutrition of the duodenum, so any injury that disrupts this circulation may produce duodenal necrosis.

The splenic artery and vein run along the posterior, superior surface of the pancreas. The artery gives rise to many small branches to the gland, and the vein receives many small tributaries. These multiple, short vessels make dissection difficult. The tail of the pancreas lies within the splenic pedicle and is easily injured during splenectomy.

The uncinate process is the posterior extension of the head of the pancreas. The superior mesenteric artery and vein course side by side along the uncinate process, deep to the pancreas. Small arterial branches and venous tributaries connect these vessels to the posterior aspect of the pancreas.

The liver, the largest organ in the abdomen, is located in the right upper quadrant under the diaphragm. The liver has many essential roles in the metabolism of absorbed nutrients: synthesis of proteins; excretion of lipid-soluble materials, including drugs; and the production of bile, which is necessary for the absorption of lipids from the intestine.

The liver has a dual blood supply; arterial blood from the hepatic artery branch of the celiac axis and a much larger volume via the portal vein, which collects the venous blood from the stomach, spleen, intestine, and colon. The portal vein is formed by the joining of the splenic, inferior mesenteric, and superior mesenteric veins posterior and superior to the pancreas. The portal vein branches within the liver to distribute its flow to both lobes and to their segments. The blood leaves the liver to enter the inferior vena cava via the hepatic veins.

The bile formed in the liver is carried by the intrahepatic bile ducts, which coalesce to form the common hepatic duct. The common hepatic duct is joined by the cystic duct to become the common bile duct. The common bile duct passes posteriorly, behind the duodenum, to traverse the head of the pancreas and enter the duodenum through the ampulla of Vater. The main pancreatic duct (Wirsung) also enters the duodenum at this point, either adjacent to the common bile duct or by a common channel.

The gallbladder serves as a reservoir for the bile that is secreted by the liver. It lies on the inferior surface of the liver to the right of the midline and joins the common bile duct via the cystic duct. The cystic artery, a branch of the hepatic artery, furnishes its major arterial supply. Venous drainage is by multiple, small tributaries into the liver bed, joining the portal system.

FUNCTION OF THE GASTROINTESTINAL TRACT

The primary and essential function of the gastrointestinal tract is the absorption of fluids and nutrients. Gastrointestinal secretion and motility serve to prepare the ingested materials for the absorptive process.

The alimentary tract is divided into functional segments by sphincters, which maintain a resting tone greater than the adjacent segments. The oral pharynx and respiratory pathway are separated from the esophagus by the upper esophageal sphincter, and the esophagus is protected from the irritant action of acid gastric juice by the lower esophageal sphincter. These two sphincters, in the resting state, separate the body of the esophagus from the pharynx and airways above and from the stomach below. Both relax in response to swallowing and close after the bolus has passed. The stomach is separated from the duodenum by the pyloric sphincter, which relaxes as the peristaltic wave sweeps down the stomach but allows only a small amount of gastric contents to pass into the duodenum at a time. The pylorus also prevents the reflux of bile into the stomach. Bile salts are damaging to the lining of the stomach and make it susceptible to irritant action of the acid gastric juice. The sphincter of Oddi separates the pancreatic and common bile ducts from the duodenum and prevents reflux of duodenal contents into these glands, but does relax in response to the hormone cholecystokininpancreozymin (CCK-PZ), which causes the gallbladder to contract, emptying the bile into the duodenum. The small intestine is separated from the colon by the ileocecal sphincter. This sphincter prevents the reflux of colonic contents into the small bowel, an important function because contamination of the small intestine with colonic bacteria interferes with its absorptive function. And, finally, the anal sphincters provide control over defecation.

The preparation of food for absorption begins in the mouth, where it is physically broken up by chewing. Digestion of starch is initiated by salivary amylase, which continues until the ingested food is acidified in the stomach. In the stomach, the emulsification process is continued by the churning action of gastric peristaltic waves. In addition, the stomach secretes hydrochloric acid and the protein-splitting enzyme pepsin, which starts the digestion of protein in preparation for its absorption. The peptic digestion of protein is not, however, an essential step in protein absorption. Gastric secretion and motility are

Plate 54.
Liver—Vascular and Biliary Systems

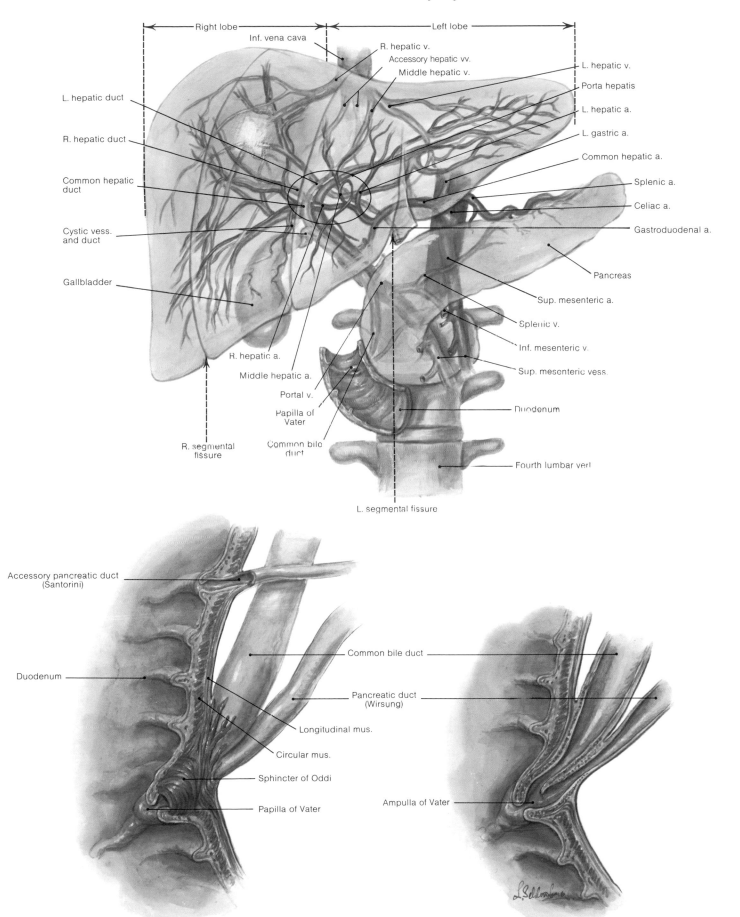

Right lobe

Left lobe

Inf. vena cava

R. hepatic v.

Accessory hepatic vv.

Middle hepatic v.

L. hepatic v.

Porta hepatis

L. hepatic a.

L. hepatic duct

R. hepatic duct

L. gastric a.

Common hepatic a.

Common hepatic duct

Splenic a.

Celiac a.

Cystic vess. and duct

Gastroduodenal a.

Gallbladder

Pancreas

R. hepatic a.

Sup. mesenteric a.

Middle hepatic a.

Splenic v.

Inf. mesenteric v.

Portal v.

Sup. mesenteric vess.

Papilla of Vater

Duodenum

Common bile duct

Fourth lumbar vert.

R. segmental fissure

L. segmental fissure

Accessory pancreatic duct (Santorini)

Common bile duct

Duodenum

Pancreatic duct (Wirsung)

Longitudinal mus.

Circular mus.

Sphincter of Oddi

Papilla of Vater

Ampulla of Vater

controlled by a variety of neural and hormonal influences. The main stimulatory influences are cholinergic fibers in the vagus and the hormone gastrin, which is released from G (gastrin) cells in the antrum. Gastrin release is increased by a variety of stimuli, such as distention of the stomach, protein digestion products, and an alkaline pH in the stomach.

The motility of the stomach, pylorus, and duodenum are nicely integrated so only a small amount of liquefied gastric chyme is delivered to the duodenum at a time. The arrival of this material in the duodenum releases two hormones, secretin and CCK-PZ. Secretin causes the outpouring of a large volume of bicarbonate-rich fluid from the pancreas and, to a lesser extent, increases the flow and bicarbonate concentration of bile. CCK-PZ causes the pancreas to pour out its digestive enzymes; in addition, it causes the gallbladder to contract and the sphincter of Oddi to relax so that bile acids necessary for the solubilization of the products of fat digestion are emptied into the duodenum as the meal is arriving from the stomach. Secretin and CCK-PZ delay gastric emptying until the duodenal contents have been alkalinized to the pH for optimal action of the pancreatic enzymes. Carbohydrates are broken down to disaccharides, which are then hydrolyzed to monosaccharides by enzymes on the brush border of the intestinal cells. These monosaccharides are transported into the cell by specific carrier mechanism, and leave the intestinal mucosa and enter the general circulation via the mesenteric and portal veins. Proteins are split by proteolytic enzymes, which are secreted by the pancreas in an inactive form and are only activated through the conversion of trypsinogen to trypsin by the intestinal enzyme, enterokinase. Trypsin in turn activates the rest of the proteolytic enzymes; hence, normally the proteolytic enzymes are inactive while within the pancreas but become active as they enter the duodenum.

The products of protein digestion are peptides, which are taken into the absorbing intestinal cells, where they are split to amino acids, which then leave via the mesenteric and portal veins. Fats are digested by pancreatic lipase to fatty acids and monoglycerides. These digestion products, along with fat-soluble vitamins, are solubilized by the detergent action of bile acids and are carried to the intestinal cell, where they are absorbed. The fatty acids and monoglycerides are resynthesized, again solubilized by the incorporation into a protein envelope, the chylomicron, which leaves the cell and is carried to the general circulation via the lymphatics. Normally, this process of absorption of carbohydrates, proteins, and fats is completed before the food has gone more than one-third of the way through the small intestine. The remainder of the intestine reabsorbs most of the fluid that has entered, either ingested or secreted. The distal small intestine, the ileum, has two specific absorptive functions, first, the absorption of vitamin B_{12}. The absorption of this vitamin is dependent on being bound to intrinsic factor, which is secreted in the stomach and specific transport receptors in the ileum. Bile acids are specifically absorbed in the ileum and carried back to the liver by way of the portal blood, excreted in the bile, and stored in the gallbladder until the next meal. Normally less than 5 percent of the bile acids are lost into the colon each day.

From one to two liters of fluid are delivered to the colon per day. In the ascending and transverse colon, fluid and electrolytes are reabsorbed and the materials passed. In the descending colon, the unabsorbed food substances, primarily cellulose, desquamated cells, and colonic bacteria are made into solid mass, which is stored and evacuated through the anus by the defecation reflex one or two times a day.

Plate 55.
Colon, Rectum, and Anus—Physiology

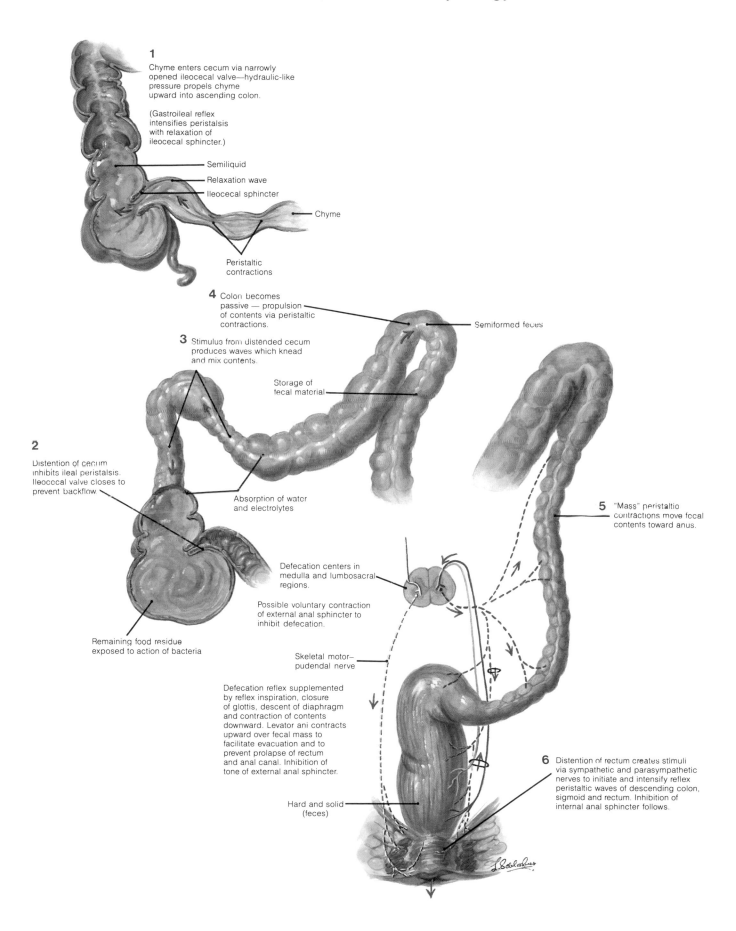

1 Chyme enters cecum via narrowly opened ileocecal valve—hydraulic-like pressure propels chyme upward into ascending colon.

(Gastroileal reflex intensifies peristalsis with relaxation of ileocecal sphincter.)

Semiliquid

Relaxation wave

Ileocecal sphincter

Chyme

Peristaltic contractions

4 Colon becomes passive — propulsion of contents via peristaltic contractions.

Semiformed feces

3 Stimulus from distended cecum produces waves which knead and mix contents.

Storage of fecal material

2 Distention of cecum inhibits ileal peristalsis. Ileocecal valve closes to prevent backflow.

Absorption of water and electrolytes

5 "Mass" peristaltic contractions move fecal contents toward anus.

Defecation centers in medulla and lumbosacral regions.

Possible voluntary contraction of external anal sphincter to inhibit defecation.

Remaining food residue exposed to action of bacteria

Skeletal motor— pudendal nerve

Defecation reflex supplemented by reflex inspiration, closure of glottis, descent of diaphragm and contraction of contents downward. Levator ani contracts upward over fecal mass to facilitate evacuation and to prevent prolapse of rectum and anal canal. Inhibition of tone of external anal sphincter.

6 Distention of rectum creates stimuli via sympathetic and parasympathetic nerves to initiate and intensify reflex peristaltic waves of descending colon, sigmoid and rectum. Inhibition of internal anal sphincter follows.

Hard and solid (feces)

The Female Generative Tract and Pregnancy

Howard W. Jones, Jr., M.D.

The female generative tract consists of the vulva, vagina, uterus, two Fallopian tubes, and two ovaries, together with their ligamentous and muscular support and vascular and nerve supply.

The greatest part of the vulva consists of two vertical outer folds of skin (the labia majora), which converge and join anteriorly with the mons veneris, a pad of tissue overlying the symphysis pubis. Two smaller vertical folds (the labia minora), located within the labia majora, surround the vaginal orifice. Anteriorly, the labia minora are continuous with the foreskin (prepuce) of the clitoris, a small organ composed of erectile tissue and homologous with the male penis. The urethral meatus is between the clitoris and the vaginal orifice.

Entering the vulva are the ducts of Skene's and Bartholin's glands, which furnish lubrication. The hymen is a rudimentary structure at the vaginal orifice.

The vagina is a potential space about 10 cm in length extending from the vulva to the uterus. The walls of the vagina consist of an inner epithelial layer, a muscular layer, and an outer elastic fibrous layer. The vagina receives semen from the male during intercourse and provides an egress for the menstrual flow and a canal for the passage of the fetus during childbirth.

The uterus is a pear-shaped organ about 10 cm in length and 6 cm in width. Its lower portion, or cervix, extends into the upper vagina for a distance of about 2 cm. The cavity of the uterus, a triangular area about 2.5 cm on a side, is continuous with the cervical canal, and by this with the vagina below and with the lumina of the Fallopian tubes above. The uterus, whose muscle wall is about 2 cm in thickness, is held in position by the broad ligaments. The lining of the uterus (endometrium) undergoes changes each month in preparation for pregnancy. In the event pregnancy does not occur, the endometrium is discharged as the menstrual flow. The fertilized ovum enters the endometrial cavity from seven to ten days after ovulation and there implants itself within the endometrium, where it grows and develops.

The Fallopian tubes, each about 10 cm in length, are held in position by the broad ligaments. Each tube consists of a narrow isthmic portion attached to the uterus, a longer ampullary portion, and a distal infundibular portion terminating in the fimbria, which collect the egg after ovulation.

The ovaries are two bodies about 3.0 by 2.5 by 2.0 cm that weigh about 10 gm. They are attached to the infundibulopelvic ligaments, which contain the ovarian vessels. At birth, each ovary contains about 200,000 developing oöcytes, of which about 200 are ovulated during menstrual life.

In addition to acting as the reservoir of genetic material for future generations, the ovary is an important endocrine gland, which produces the female sex hormone (estrogen), as well as some androgen, and progesterone from the corpus luteum, which develops from the ovarian follicle after ovulation and has a life span of about fourteen days.

INNERVATION OF THE UTERUS, CERVIX, VAGINA, BLADDER, RECTUM, AND PERINEUM

The pelvic viscera are innervated mostly by the sympathetic nervous system. However, somatic sensory and motor pathways supply the urinary and intestinal voluntary sphincters, as well as the skin and muscles of the perineum.

The anatomic arrangement of the sympathetic nerves varies widely. Retroperitoneally, a network of sympathetic fibers in front of the aorta is known as the aortic plexus. On either side of this are two main strands of nervous tissue derived from the lumbar sympathetic ganglia. These fuse with the aortic plexus in front of the fifth lumbar vertebra or thereabouts to form the superior hypogastric plexus from which courses the hypogastric (presacral) nerve.

In front of the upper part of the sacrum, the hypogastric nerve becomes the middle hypogastric plexus; it then divides into two parts around the rectum, where it becomes known as the inferior hypogastric plexus. This plexus passes forward onto the uterosacral ligament and is known as the ganglion or plexus of *Frankenhäuser,* the *lateral cervical plexus,* the *uterovaginal plexus,* or, more commonly, the *pelvic plexus.*

The pelvic plexus is made up of interlacing nerve fibers containing large numbers of small microscopic ganglia. The pelvic plexus receives fibers from the sacral sympathetic ganglia and parasympathetic fibers from the nervi erigentes. The sympathetic fibers relay in the ganglia, but the parasympathetic fibers merely pass through the cell stations to the adjacent viscera.

The parasympathetic nerves supplying the pelvic viscera (except for the ovaries and the proximal part of the tubes) arise from the anterior roots of the second, third, and fourth sacral nerves. These nerves fuse and form the nervi erigentes.

The external genitalia have a parasympathetic and sympathetic nerve supply from the same sources as the pelvic organs. The parasympathetic supply dilates the vessels to the erectile tissue and causes the bulbocavernosus and the ischiocavernosus muscles to contract with sexual orgasm.

Somatic sensory branches to the skin of the perineum, including parts of the external genitalia and motor branches to the muscles of the perineum, are derived from the pudendal and ilioinguinal nerves.

The innervation of the uterus is a subject of some controversy. Apparently the uterus has a sympathetic supply from the hypogastric nerve and a parasympathetic supply from the sacral plexus. The sympathetic supply seems to be responsible for controlling the circular muscular fibers around the cervix.

Sensory fibers pass to the spinal cord from the uterus through the presacral nerve. Presacral sympathectomy severs these pain-conducting fibers, useful for the relief of spasmodic dysmenorrhea and resulting in a painless first stage of labor.

The Fallopian tubes are innervated peripherally by sympathetic fibers from the ovarian plexus and medially by sympathetic fibers derived from the pelvic plexus. The parasympathetic supply is derived from the vagus via the ovarian plexus.

Both the sympathetic and parasympathetic fibers to the ovary reach the ovary by way of the ovarian plexus.

The bladder has a sympathetic supply from the hypogastric nerves and a parasympathetic supply through the nervi erigentes.

The anatomy of the pelvic floor is shown in chapter 21, in association with the perineum and male genitourinary system.

PREGNANCY

After fertilization, which takes place in the Fallopian tube, the early embryo enters the uterine cavity and buries itself into the endomentrium, where it first develops. All organs of the embryo develop from the three primary germ layers (ectoderm, mesoderm, and endoderm), which form early in the embryo. From the ectoderm are derived the nervous system and sense organs, the epidermis, brain, and spinal cord. From the mesoderm are derived the skeletal, muscular, circulatory, and some parts of the reproductive system and the kidneys, ureters, and other structures; and from the endoderm are derived the alimentary canal and its derivatives, such as the respiratory system, thyroid, pancreas, liver, gallbladder, and parts of the reproductive organs.

During pregnancy, the uterus gradually rises in the abdomen, until near the end of pregnancy it reaches almost to the xiphoid. Before labor, the head drops lower into the pelvis, and the fundus of the uterus, prior to labor, may be somewhat lower than previously.

A great variety of fetal abnormalities occur, some of which are genetic, others environmental, but much remains to be learned about this aspect of human development. However, certain types of genetic defects can be ascertained during embryonic life. This can be done by the examination of cells removed with a small amount of amniotic fluid at about the sixteenth week of gestation. The cells in the amniotic sac are of fetal origin, and after they have been cultured they may be examined for chromosomal content and certain biochemical constituents, abnormalities of which reflect the diseased state of the fetus. At the present time, the only method of control is termination of the pregnancy of seriously handicapped children, e.g., those affected with Down's syndrome (47, XX, +G21 or 47, XY, +G21) or Tay-Sachs disease, a very serious disorder due to an enzymatic deficiency inherited as an autosomal recessive.

At term, labor is initiated by a mechanism as yet unknown. During the first stage of labor, uterine contractions press the presenting part, usually the head, into the cervix as the cervical canal dilates.

During the second stage of labor, uterine contractions become more frequent and painful, and at this stage the abdominal muscles by voluntary action may aid in propelling the fetus through the vagina. Immediately after birth, the umbilical cord can be ligated and severed.

In the third stage of labor, the placenta is expelled. With the delivery of the child and the placenta, the uterus contracts and thereby stops the bleeding that would otherwise occur. Contractions of the uterus may be slightly painful for several days and are known as *afterpains.*

Plate 56.
Genitourinary Tract, Female

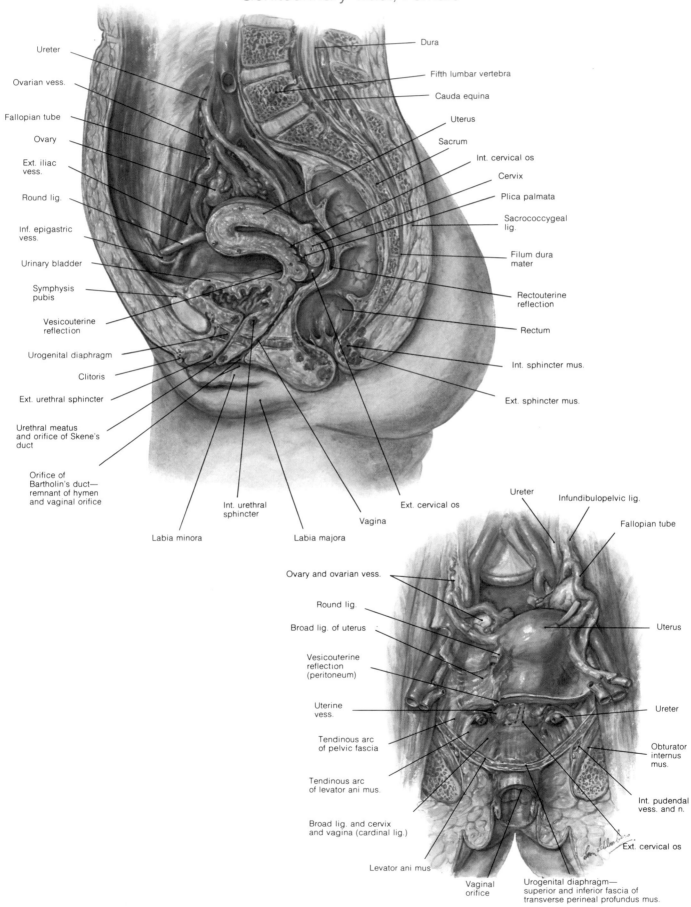

Ureter

Ovarian vess.

Fallopian tube

Ovary

Ext. iliac
vess.

Round lig.

Inf. epigastric
vess.

Urinary bladder

Symphysis
pubis

Vesicouterine
reflection

Urogenital diaphragm

Clitoris

Ext. urethral sphincter

Urethral meatus
and orifice of Skene's
duct

Orifice of
Bartholin's duct—
remnant of hymen
and vaginal orifice

Int. urethral
sphincter

Labia minora

Labia majora

Vagina

Ext. cervical os

Dura

Fifth lumbar vertebra

Cauda equina

Uterus

Sacrum

Int. cervical os

Cervix

Plica palmata

Sacrococcygeal
lig.

Filum dura
mater

Rectouterine
reflection

Rectum

Int. sphincter mus.

Ext. sphincter mus.

Ovary and ovarian vess.

Round lig.

Broad lig. of uterus

Vesicouterine
reflection
(peritoneum)

Uterine
vess.

Tendinous arc
of pelvic fascia

Tendinous arc
of levator ani mus.

Broad lig. and cervix
and vagina (cardinal lig.)

Levator ani mus

Vaginal
orifice

Ureter

Infundibulopelvic lig.

Fallopian tube

Uterus

Ureter

Obturator
internus
mus.

Int. pudendal
vess. and n.

Ext. cervical os

Urogenital diaphragm—
superior and inferior fascia of
transverse perineal profundus mus.

Plate 57.
Genitourinary Innervation of the Uterus, Cervix, Vagina, Bladder, Rectum, and Perineum

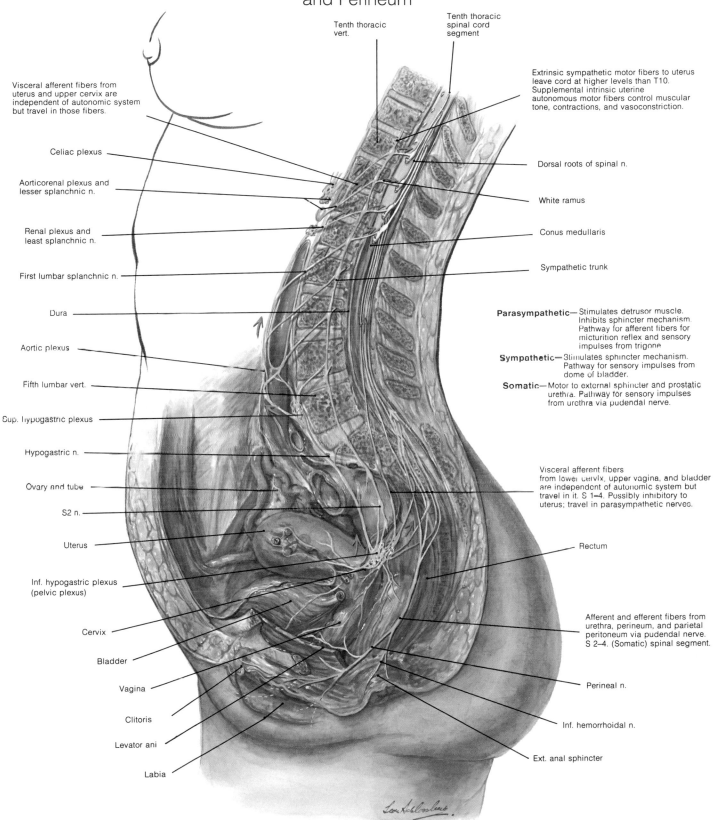

Tenth thoracic vert.

Tenth thoracic spinal cord segment

Visceral afferent fibers from uterus and upper cervix are independent of autonomic system but travel in those fibers.

Extrinsic sympathetic motor fibers to uterus leave cord at higher levels than T10. Supplemental intrinsic uterine autonomous motor fibers control muscular tone, contractions, and vasoconstriction.

Celiac plexus

Dorsal roots of spinal n.

Aorticorenal plexus and lesser splanchnic n.

White ramus

Renal plexus and least splanchnic n.

Conus medullaris

First lumbar splanchnic n.

Sympathetic trunk

Dura

Parasympathetic—Stimulates detrusor muscle. Inhibits sphincter mechanism. Pathway for afferent fibers for micturition reflex and sensory impulses from trigone.

Aortic plexus

Sympathetic—Stimulates sphincter mechanism. Pathway for sensory impulses from dome of bladder.

Fifth lumbar vert.

Somatic—Motor to external sphincter and prostatic urethra. Pathway for sensory impulses from urethra via pudendal nerve.

Sup. hypogastric plexus

Hypogastric n.

Visceral afferent fibers from lower cervix, upper vagina, and bladder are independent of autonomic system but travel in it. S 1–4. Possibly inhibitory to uterus; travel in parasympathetic nerves.

Ovary and tube

S2 n.

Uterus

Rectum

Inf. hypogastric plexus (pelvic plexus)

Afferent and efferent fibers from urethra, perineum, and parietal peritoneum via pudendal nerve. S 2–4. (Somatic) spinal segment.

Cervix

Bladder

Vagina

Perineal n.

Clitoris

Inf. hemorrhoidal n.

Levator ani

Ext. anal sphincter

Labia

Plate 58.
Pregnancy

PREGNANCY AT 16 WEEKS

Uterus

Placenta

Site for amniocentesis
for detection of genetic
defects

Fetus

Amniotic
fluid

Cervix

PREGNANCY AT TERM

After dropping

9
8
7
6
5
4
3rd
month

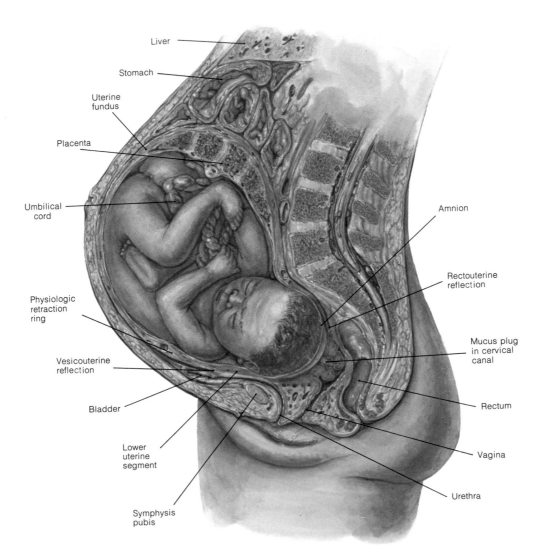

Liver

Stomach

Uterine
fundus

Placenta

Umbilical
cord

Physiologic
retraction
ring

Vesicouterine
reflection

Bladder

Lower
uterine
segment

Symphysis
pubis

Amnion

Rectouterine
reflection

Mucus plug
in cervical
canal

Rectum

Vagina

Urethra

PREGNANCY AT TERM

The Menstrual Cycle

H. Lorrin Lau, M.D.

The term *menstruation* refers to the monthly shedding of endometrium from the uterus, whereas the term *human menstrual cycle* refers to a recurring series of events in the hypothalamic-pituitary-ovarian-uterine axis responsible for ovulation and reproduction.

Day 1 of the cycle is the first day of bleeding.

Changes in geophysical location; influences such as light, smell, and sound; and emotional stress such as death in the family or the stress of college examinations can seriously disturb the rhythm of the cycle or cause a period of amenorrhea. These external stimuli act presumably via the cortex to the hypothalamus.

The hypothalamus produces releasing factors (peptides of MW 2000) for follicle-stimulating hormone (FSH), luteinizing hormone (LH), and a prolactin-inhibiting factor (PF). These are carried by the hypophyseal portal capillary network to the anterior pituitary, where the release of FSH and LH is stimulated but that of prolactin is inhibited. This initiates the follicular phase, in which there is growth of the Graafian follicle, proliferation of endometrium, rises in serum FSH and LH, and increased secretion by the theca interna of 17 α-hydroxyprogesterone, androstenedione, and estradiol. Steroidal contraceptives such as norethynodrel with mestranol (Enovid) act on the hypothalamus by depressing the releasing factors.

At midcycle, or the ovulatory phase, which is day 14 in the idealized cycle, LH induces final maturation of the follicle ripened by FSH and expulsion of the egg from the surface of the ovary. FSH and LH show their largest spike at this time (day 14); a smaller spike of FSH occurs in the follicular phase in many cycles. The space left by the egg becomes a corpus luteum (yellow body), which secretes progesterone, the steroid that resets the hypothalamic thermostat to give the typical elevation in the pattern of basal body temperature. Other steroids such as estradiol and 17 α-hydroxyprogesterone rise concomitantly with the LH peak. By contrast, FSH alone does not stimulate the production of steroids.

The life span of the corpus luteum is about fourteen days, determines the duration of the secretory phase, and is affected by luteotrophic and luteolytic agents. LH is definitely luteotrophic in man, while prolactin may also be luteotrophic. In sheep, prostaglandins (lipid-soluble, unsaturated hydroxy acids with 20 carbons) are definitely luteolytic, while in man their luteolytic activity is still being studied.

The uterus reflects the steroidal activity of the ovary. In the proliferative phase, marked mitotic activity is seen in the glands and stroma with straight narrow glands containing basal nuclei and pseudostratification. At ovulation, these decrease. After ovulation basal vacuoles appears in the apex of the glands, which enlarge and acquire a sawtooth appearance, with ragged edges, where secretion is discharged into the lumen. The stroma swells and spiral arteries become prominent. Two days prior to menstruation, the corpus luteum regresses to induce disappearance of the stroma swelling, spasm of the arteries, and a filling with material of the glands, which show an irregular apex and single round basal nuclei without stratification.

The vaginal epithelium, thickened at ovulation with cornified cells, decreases in height and shows precornified cells.

Spasm of the spiral arteries, hypoxia of the endometrium, and the appearance of sheets of predecidual cells initiate sloughing of the uterine epithelium (*menses*), and another cycle begins.

Plate 59.
The Menstrual Cycle

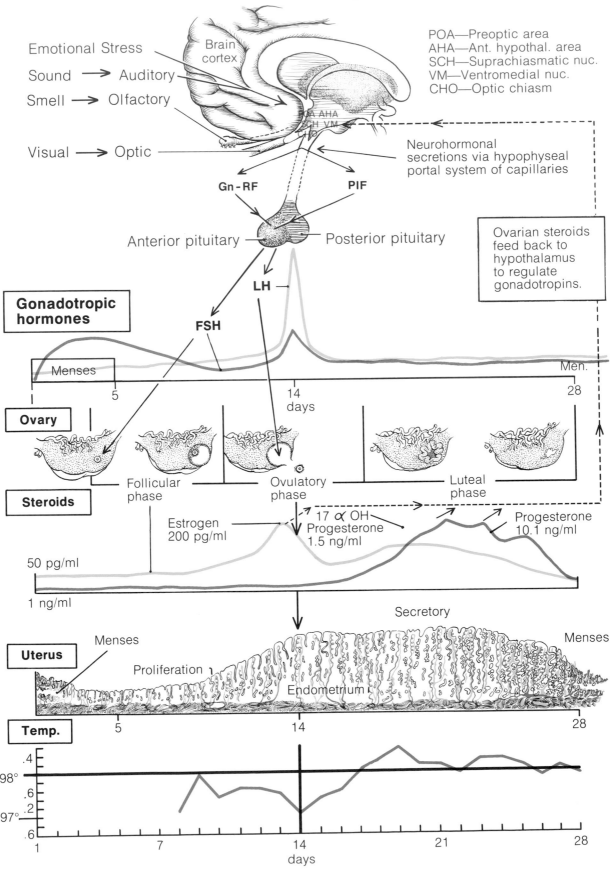

Emotional Stress

Sound → Auditory

Smell → Olfactory

Visual → Optic

Brain cortex

POA—Preoptic area
AHA—Ant. hypothal. area
SCH—Suprachiasmatic nuc.
VM—Ventromedial nuc.
CHO—Optic chiasm

Neurohormonal secretions via hypophyseal portal system of capillaries

Gn - RF   PIF

Anterior pituitary   Posterior pituitary

Ovarian steroids feed back to hypothalamus to regulate gonadotropins.

LH →

Gonadotropic hormones

FSH

Menses   Men.

5   14
days   28

Ovary

Follicular phase   Ovulatory phase   Luteal phase

Steroids

Estrogen 200 pg/ml   17 α OH Progesterone 1.5 ng/ml   Progesterone 10.1 ng/ml

50 pg/ml

1 ng/ml

Secretory

Uterus   Menses   Menses

Proliferation   Endometrium

5   14   28

Temp.

.4
98°
.6
.2
97°
.6

1   7   14   21   28
days

21

The Kidneys, Male Genitourinary System, and Perineum

Rainer M. E. Engel, M.D.

The normal urinary tract consists of two kidneys, two ureters, a bladder, and a urethra. Except for the urethra, the urinary tract is essentially the same in both males and females. The function of the urinary tract consists of maintenance of fluid and electrolyte balance, which is achieved by secreting water and various waste products of the body. A number of substances are conserved by reabsorption in the kidney. Others are excreted, and the final end product, urine, is delivered into the collecting system.

The kidneys are paired organs, each approximately 11 cm long and 6 cm wide, that lie in the retroperitoneal area at the level of the lower thoracic and upper lumbar vertebrae. The right is usually somewhat lower. The upper pole borders on the diaphragm, and the lower portion extends over the iliopsoas muscle. The posterior surface is protected in its upper part by the lower ribs. The renal tissue is covered by the renal capsule and surrounded by Gerota's fascia, which is quite firm and will usually confine blood and urine extravasations as well as suppurative processes. Medially, blood vessels, lymphatics, and nerves enter each kidney at its midportion, the hilum. Behind the blood vessels, the renal pelvis, with the ureter, leaves the kidney. Blood enters the kidney through the renal artery, which is usually single, and which branches into smaller vessels supplying the different lobes of the kidney. The kidneys receive about one-fourth of the cardiac output per minute. Once the artery has entered the renal substance, it branches along the boundary between cortex and medulla and from there radiates into the parenchyma. There are no communications between the capillaries or larger vessels of the kidney. The arcuate arteries supply the cortex and give off small arterioles that form multiple convoluted tufts, the glomeruli. From each glomerulus the efferent, still arteriolar vessel leaves again to supply, with a fine network, the renal tubule of its corresponding glomerulus. These peritubular arteries empty through small venules into larger collecting veins and finally, through the renal vein, into the vena cava. The left renal vein is longer than the right, as it crosses the aorta to reach the vena cava, and receives the left gonadal vein. The right gonadal (ovarian or spermatic) vein empties separately, below the renal vein, into the vena cava.

Numerous lymphatic channels are found throughout the kidney. These drain into hilar nodes, which communicate with periaortic nodes above and below the hilar area. Cross communications to the contralateral side have also been demonstrated.

Urine is filtered by the glomerulus and collected into a space confined by Bowman's capsule. From there it is transported through the proximal convoluted tubule, Henle's loop, and distal convoluted tubule into the collecting tubules that empty through the pyramid of the medulla into the caliceal cups. Urine is filtered mainly by the hydrostatic pressure of the blood pressure. Thus, when the blood pressure drops, filtration will also stop and urine formation ceases. Other factors important in the formation of urine are: (1) the osmotic pressure, which is largely produced by the plasma protein in the blood; and (2) the back pressure of already excreted urine in the collecting system. The glomerulus acts, in other words, like a sieve that will strain corpuscles and will also hold back protein. This glomerular filtration would allow approximately 190 liters of fluid to be excreted daily. However, as the filtrate passes from the glomerulus into Bowman's capsule and into the tubules, reabsorption, secretion, and excretion will alter the final end product. Only about 1 percent of the total filtrate will be excreted as urine into the renal pelvis.

Hormones play an active role in the reabsorption of both water and other substances. Antidiuretic hormone (ADH) regulates absorption and elimination of water, depending on the needs of the body. Aldosterone promotes reabsorption of sodium and excretion of potassium. Parathyroid hormone increases the reabsorption of calcium and decreases the reabsorption of phosphorus.

The amount of functioning renal tissue is fortunately far in excess of the minimum requirements for life. About one-third of the normal tissue will adequately, and without appreciable alteration of function tests, sustain life and growth.

After urine has entered the collecting system, it remains unchanged. The urine is collected in the renal pelvis and moves, by peristaltic waves, across the ureteropelvic junction and through the ureter. One of the common sites of obstruction of kidneys is at the level of the ureteropelvic junction. The blood supply to the ureter is derived from numerous areas. Fine branches having their origin from the renal blood vessels supply the ureter from the renal pelvis. The lower portion receives its blood supply from vesical arteries, and the midportion is supplied by branches from the lumbar vessels. The lymphatics drain into the areas that correspond to the arterial supply, and veins show a similar distribution. The ureters enters the bladder through a long tunnel through the muscular wall of the bladder and the mucosa. Each ureteral orifice is a small slitlike opening. The ureters usually lie about 2 to 3 cm apart in the adult and are situated slightly off the midline, about 2 cm above the internal opening of the urethra. The area between these three openings is called the *trigone*. Under normal conditions, urine will pass through the ureteral orifice only in one direction, i.e., into the bladder. As the bladder pressure increases, the mucosal tissue over the inner wall of the ureter will be pressed against the back wall of the ureter, thus preventing backing up of urine, or vesicoureteral reflux. As the ureter passes from the kidney into the bladder, it encounters three narrow points. The first is at the ureteropelvic junction; the second, at its crossing with the iliac vessels; and the third, where it penetrates the bladder wall. Stones, during their passage from the kidney down into the bladder, may lodge at one of these three points and produce obstruction.

The bladder is a rounded, hollow muscular organ that normally distends to hold an average of 500 ml. However, under certain conditions, the bladder can be distended much beyond this capacity. In the male, the posterior surface of the bladder is in proximity to the rectum. In the female, the superior part of the vagina and the uterus are interposed between the bladder and rectum. The dome of the bladder is covered by peritoneum.

The bladder receives its blood supply from branches of the internal iliac or hypogastric arteries, with smaller branches from the hemorrhoidal and uterine arteries. Lymphatic drainage, which is important in the spread of bladder cancers, follows the internal, external, and common iliac vessels predominantly.

The nerve supply to the bladder includes the parasympathetic system, which supplies the detrusor muscle, which will contract the bladder; the sympathetic branch of the autonomic system supplies the base of the bladder. The pudendal nerve supplies the external sphincter, which surrounds the urethra. Connections, or synapses, between these various nerve supplies allow for simultaneous contraction of the detrusor, and relaxation and opening of internal and external sphincters. Sensory fibers that transmit both filling and stretch sensation of the distended bladder are carried through parasympathetic fibers to the spinal cord, where the primary reflex center for the bladder is located at the level of S2 to S4. A reflex arc may, at this level, permit some form of function of the bladder in certain patients with spinal cord injuries. Tracts in the spinal cord connect the primary center with higher centers that allow us to suppress the urge to void and become "toilet-trained." Thus, the normal bladder will continue to fill without causing us discomfort, and at its usual filling limit will elicit nervous stimuli that we, however, can override, to expand the capacity and empty the bladder at our convenience.

The ureters will permit transport of urine into the bladder. Even with complete filling of the bladder, there will be no incontinence of urine. Once the act of voiding or micturition begins, the bladder will empty to completion.

Urine leaves the bladder through the urethra. In the female, this is a fairly short tubular organ about 3 to 5 cm long with its external opening between the labia minora; it courses along the anterior vault of the vagina. The male urethra is an S-shaped, tubular organ, approximately 20 cm long. At its beginning, it runs through the prostate, a secondary sex gland. The prostatic urethra is 2.5 to 3.0 cm long. Just below the prostate, the urethra pierces the pelvic diaphragm, an area in which it is almost immobile and not very distensible. This diaphragmatic portion of the urethra is also called the *membranous urethra,* and is approximately 1 cm long. Below this, the bulbus urethra, a patulous part of the urethra, begins, and, following this, the channel tapers at the penoscrotal junction into the pendulous urethra, which lies in the ventral wall of the penis and is on its ventral surface, covered by the corpus spongiosum.

The bladder neck is the most common site of obstruction of the urinary tract in the male. Usually this is produced by prostatic enlargement, due to benign

Plate 60.
Genitourinary Tract, Male

Puboprostatic lig.

Ant. peritoneal reflection

Int. urethral sphincter

Vas deferens

Ureteral orifice

Ureter

Seminal vesicle

Medial umbilical lig.

Space of Retzius (fat pad)

Scarpa's fascia

Post. peritoneal reflection (rectovesical peritoneal pouch)

Ext. urethral sphincter and urogenital diaphragm

Littre's gland

Buck's fascia

Corpus cavernosum penis

Corpus cavernosum urethra

Dartos

Colles' fascia

Glans penis

Prepuce

Testis

Ejaculatory duct

Denonvilliers' fascia

Rectum

Prostate

Scrotum

Central tendon

Cowper's gland

Rectourethralis mus.

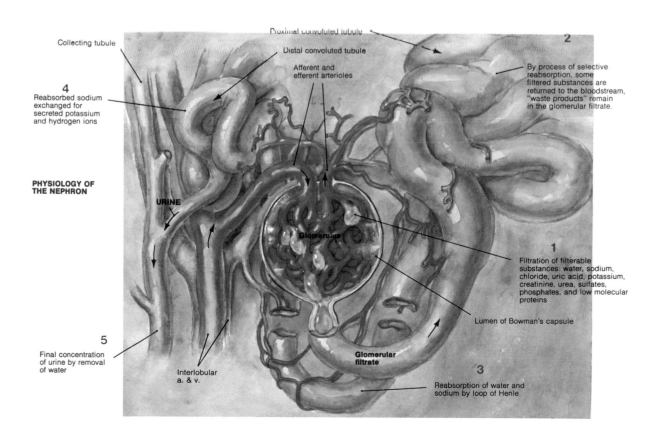

Collecting tubule

Proximal convoluted tubule

Distal convoluted tubule

Afferent and efferent arterioles

2

By process of selective reabsorption, some filtered substances are returned to the bloodstream, "waste products" remain in the glomerular filtrate.

4
Reabsorbed sodium exchanged for secreted potassium and hydrogen ions

PHYSIOLOGY OF THE NEPHRON

URINE

Glomerulus

1

Filtration of filterable substances: water, sodium, chloride, uric acid, potassium, creatinine, urea, sulfates, phosphates, and low molecular proteins

Lumen of Bowman's capsule

5
Final concentration of urine by removal of water

Interlobular a. & v.

Glomerular filtrate

3

Reabsorption of water and sodium by loop of Henle

Plate 61.
Genitourinary Tract, Male—Vessels and Nerves

Sympathetic trunk and greater splanchnic n.

Diaphragm

Inf. vena cava

Adrenal gland, vess., and nn.

Renal vess. and nerve plexus

Testicular vess. and n.

Aorta

Iliohypogastric n.

Ilioinguinal n.

Lateral femoral cutaneous n.

Genitofemoral n.

Lumboinguinal n.

Ext. spermatic n.

Bladder and ureteral orifice

Femoral vessels

Prostate and orifices of ejaculatory ducts on verumontanum

Corpus cavernosum urethra

Corpus cavernosum penis

Cutaneous v. of penis and dorsal vess. and n.

Esophagus

Vagus nn.

Lesser and least splanchnic nn.

Celiac plexus of nerves and sup. mesenteric a. (parasympathetic)

Celiac ganglion (sympathetic) aorticorenal ganglion

Pelvis of kidney

Kidney

Cortex

Medulla

Major calyx

Minor calyx

L. testicular v.

Ureteropelvic junction

Ureter and n.

Common iliac vess.

Sup. hypogastric plexus

L. hypogastric n.

Pelvic nerves (parasympathetic)

Pudendal n. (somatic)

Ilioinguinal n.

Inf. hypogastric plexus

Vas deferens and seminal vesicle

Santorini plexus of vv.

Urogenital diaphragm

Testicular n.

Perineal vess. and n.

Epididymis and vas deferens

Testis

or malignant processes. As the prostate enlarges, it not only grows toward the outside perimeter but also compresses the lumen of the urethra. In benign prostatic enlargement, the small periurethral glands enlarge to form an adenoma. This can be removed by different types of prostatectomies; the true prostatic tissue in these operations is left intact. The true prostatic glands also empty into the prostatic urethra, via a dozen small ducts, into the area of the verumontanum. The two ejaculatory ducts also open into this area. The paired Cowper's glands secrete a small amount of fluid, which enters the urethra at the pelvic diaphragm. Scattered along the remainder of the urethra are the numerous small glands of Littre. Occasionally they harbor infection.

The male genital tract comprises the testes and epididymides, which lie in the scrotum and lead into the vas deferens. The vas deferens is a tube-like structure that passes through the inguinal ring, lateral to and then behind the bladder, where, after forming the ampulla, it joins with a small duct from the seminal vesicle into the ejaculatory duct.

The ejaculatory duct traverses the prostate and opens into the prostatic urethra. During delivery of the ejaculate, the combined secretion of the testes, seminal vesicles, and prostate is propelled through the urethra. At the time of ejaculation, the bladder neck stays closed, the external sphincter opens, and thus the ejaculate is propelled outwards. In patients who have undergone a prostatectomy or resection of the bladder neck, the area of least resistance is toward the bladder, and they therefore may experience a dry ejaculation or retrograde ejaculation into the bladder.

The blood supply to the testis comes from the testicular artery, which orginates on the left side from the renal artery and on the right side directly from the aorta just below the renal artery. The high origin of these vessels is explained by the embryologic origin of the testes in this area. Incomplete descent can lead to intraabdominal retention of the testis. Venous drainage occurs along the spermatic veins, which parallel the arteries.

The function of the testes is twofold: (1) they produce the male hormone, testosterone; and (2) they produce spermatozoa, which travel from the tubules of the testes into the epididymis, where they undergo maturation. From there, they are delivered into the vas deferens. Thus, a vasectomy will only interrupt delivery of spermatozoa. The bulk of the ejaculate is comprised of the fluid of the secondary sex glands, i.e., the seminal vesicle and prostate. This is not affected by vasectomy.

The urethra thus serves a twofold purpose, i.e., as a passageway for both urine and the ejaculate.

Erection of the penis is achieved through filling of the three expansile bodies of the penis with blood. These include the corpus spongiosum, which is on the undersurface of the urethra, and the paired large corpora cavernosa, which are anchored at the pubic rami and receive their blood supply from the pudendal arteries. Under erogenous stimulation, the outflow of these bodies is partially closed, and the resultant infusion of blood produces the necessary rigidity. This stimulation is mediated through branches of the sympathetic and parasympathetic nervous system, although most of the stimulation is of cerebral origin. The seminal vesicles and the prostate gland deliver fluid that contains nutrients and improves the motility of the spermatozoa. Of these, the most important is the prostate. Its blood supply is derived from branches of the inferior vesicle artery, and it drains into a rich plexus of veins, the most important of which is the plexus of Santorini, on the anterior surface of the prostate.

The anatomy of the male and female perineum and pelvic floor is shown in plate 62. Of interest is the course of the internal pudendal nerve which exits from Alcock's canal where it can be anesthetized in an effort to decrease urinary outflow resistance in patients with neurogenic imbalance between the detrusor and the musculature of the external urethral sphincter. More permanent interruption of function can be achieved by removing a portion of the middle branch, leaving intact the nerve supply to the anal sphincter and penis.

The portion of the top drawing showing dissection of the penis serves to illustrate how it is possible to separate the spongiosum from the corpora cavernosa, an anatomical fact that is helpful in partial amputation of the penis for cancer.

Plate 62.
Perineum, Male and Female

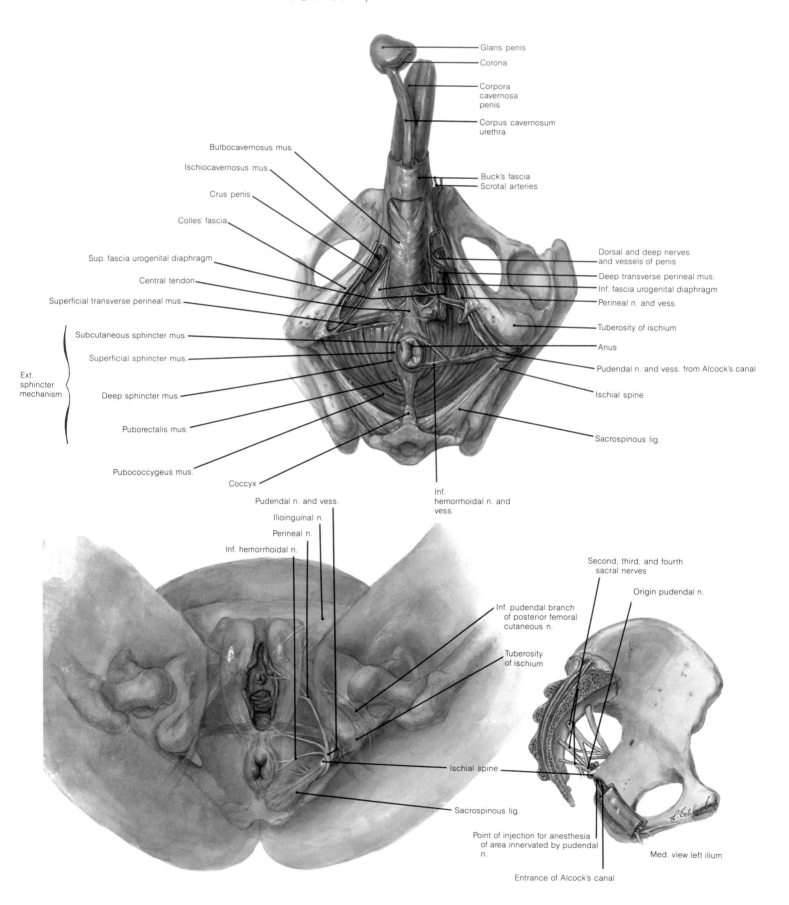

Glans penis

Corona

Corpora cavernosa penis

Corpus cavernosum urethra

Bulbocavernosus mus.

Ischiocavernosus mus.

Crus penis

Colles' fascia

Buck's fascia
Scrotal arteries

Sup. fascia urogenital diaphragm

Central tendon

Superficial transverse perineal mus.

Dorsal and deep nerves and vessels of penis

Deep transverse perineal mus.

Inf. fascia urogenital diaphragm

Perineal n. and vess.

Subcutaneous sphincter mus.

Superficial sphincter mus.

Ext. sphincter mechanism

Tuberosity of ischium

Anus

Pudendal n. and vess. from Alcock's canal

Deep sphincter mus.

Ischial spine

Puborectalis mus.

Sacrospinous lig.

Pubococcygeus mus.

Coccyx

Inf. hemorrhoidal n. and vess.

Pudendal n. and vess.

Ilioinguinal n.

Perineal n.

Inf. hemorrhoidal n.

Second, third, and fourth sacral nerves

Origin pudendal n.

Inf. pudendal branch of posterior femoral cutaneous n.

Tuberosity of ischium

Ischial spine

Sacrospinous lig.

Point of injection for anesthesia of area innervated by pudendal n.

Entrance of Alcock's canal

Med. view left ilium

The Skin

22

James J. Ryan, M.D.

The largest organ of the body, the skin, is best understood in terms of its principal function as an interface between the internal and external world. The regulation of the internal environment by detection of, protection from, and adaptation to the surrounding environment is clearly reflected in the functional anatomy of the skin. There are two types of skin: hair-bearing, covering the vast majority of the body surface; and hairless, confined to the soles of the feet and the palms of the hands. The difference in the two is simply the presence or absence of the pilosebaceous apparatus, the hair follicle and the accompanying sebaceous gland. In thickness, three major tissue layers are identified. The uppermost is a thin, stratified epithelium, the epidermis. Beneath the epidermis is the dense, fibroelastic connective tissue stroma called the *dermis* or *corium*. The third layer of the skin is the subcutaneous tissue composed of areolar and fatty connective tissue.

The epidermis or cellular investment of the entire organism consists of two principal divisions: an upper, thick keratin layer of packed cells without nuclei, the stratum corneum, and an underlying layer of nuclear cells, the stratum Malpighii, histologically divided into three layers of progressive nuclear degeneration—the stratum germinativum, stratum spinosum, and stratum granulosum. Two types of cells are present in the stratum germinativum, keratinocytes and melanocytes.

The former are most numerous and, as they differentiate and migrate upward, form the stratum corneum, which is renewed on an average of every twenty-six days. The melanocytes form the pigment granules, which are transferred to the keratinocyte cells and give the skin its color and much of its protection from intense light. The importance of the stratum corneum is to limit permeability of the skin to water and ions.

The dermis, a complex material predominantly composed of collagen and elastic fibers and diffuse ground substance, encloses cellular systems of nerves, vessels, glands, and appendages. There is a vast three-dimensional network of blood vessels, predominantly concerned with thermal regulation, seen as the subdermal vascular plexus, a dermal vascular plexus, and a subpapillary vascular plexus. The glands are the sweat glands, which provide a powerful physiologic mechanism for heat loss. The 2 to 3 million exocrine sweat glands distributed over the entire body surface are capable of delivering 2 to 3 kg of watery sweat per hour. A second type of sweat gland, the apocrine gland, occurs principally in the axilla, and is most responsive to nervous stimulation. The third gland is the sebaceous gland seen emptying into the shaft of the hair follicle and thus forming a part of the combined pilosebaceous apparatus. The skin surface lipids are largely derived from the sebum, serving to lubricate the skin and possibly influence its bacterial flora.

The subcutaneous tissue is principally adipose tissue, varying greatly in thickness over different areas of the body. This insulates underlying tissues from extremes of environmental heat or cold, as well as providing a substantial cushion. Strands of collagen extending from the dermis through the subcutaneous tissue to underlying muscle, fascial, or bony periosteal attachment influence the mobility of the skin. In the subcutaneous and dermal areas innumerable free and encapsulated nerve endings provide sensory input of many forms from the body surface.

121

Plate 63.
The Skin

Bare nerve endings (pain)

St. corneum

Subpapillary vascular plexus

Dermal vascular plexus

Int. root sheath

Ext. root sheath

Hair follicle

Hair bulb with papilla

Sympathetic n.

Blood vess.

Hair shaft

Sebaceous gland provides oil component for bacterial flora—prevents dryness.

Hair shaft

Arrector pili (smooth mus.)

Contracts when cold and elevates hair. Presses on sebaceous gland to lubricate hair.

Epidermis

Protection: Barrier to bacterial invasion. Protects deeper tissues from injury. Contains nerves to record conditions of external environment.

Heat regulation Limited excretory and absorbing powers

Corium or dermis

Sweat gland

Subcutaneous

Protective padding and storage of fat

Meissner's corpuscle (light touch)

Vascular papilla

St. corneum

St. lucidum

St. granulosum

St. spinosum

St. germinativum

Krause's end bulb (cold)

Fascia

Muscle

Vater-Pacini corpuscle (pressure)

Ruffini's corpuscle (heat)

THE SKIN (HAIRY)

Surface cells of epidermis, subject to wear and injury, are shed and are replaced by migratory cells going through stages of evolution from st. germinativum layer.

Opening of sweat gland

Duct

Ampulla of sweat gland

THE SKIN (HAIRLESS) —SOLE OF FOOT, PALM OF HAND

Glossary

Abduction Movement away from the body in the frontal plane.

Adduction Opposite of abduction, i.e., movement toward the body in the frontal plane.

Afferent Direction of entrance to a given locus, in contrast to an efferent pathway, which departs the same locus. A nerve impulse originating in the brain or a peripheral organ. An arteriole entering a tuft of capillaries (glomerulus), contrasted with the efferent arteriole, leaving the glomerulus.

Anastomosis A connection point between two separate structures; restoration of the continuity of a structure (by sutures or staples) after sectioning by trauma or surgery: blood vessel, ureter, urethra, arteriovenous fistula. Construction of a bypass to circumvent a dysfunctional site or process.

Aponeurosis Strong, fibrous, broad, flat tendon of muscle.

Appendicular Pertaining to a subordinate part of a principal structure. The appendage of an organ, e.g., atrial appendage of the heart, vermiform appendix of the intestinal tract.

Aqueduct A channel within the cerebrospinal, auditory, and vestibular systems containing an aqueous fluid. May also transmit very small blood vessels.

Arrector pili Muscles that move hair shafts and hair follicles more perpendicular to the plane of skin surface, an involuntary action associated with "goose" flesh.

Arteriole Small blood vessel, with muscular tissue, in the vessel wall.

Artery Large blood vessel with muscular tissue in the vessel wall.

Articulation Connections or mechanism of an immovable, slightly movable, or movable bony joint.

Auditory Pertaining to hearing.

Axial The long direction of a structure, such as femur, tooth, etc.

Axon Central component of a nerve fiber.

Biceps Having two heads, denoting especially certain muscles.

Bicuspid Having two cusps, or two points.

Bifid Separated into two parts.

Bifurcate Having two branches.

Bolus Refers to a mass of food being swallowed; also a mass being propelled through the intestines by peristalsis.

Brachial Pertaining to the upper arm.

Brevis Short.

Bursa Fluid-filled sac placed between or beneath movable structures (muscles, bones, tendons) to prevent friction during movement.

Calyx A cup-shaped extension of the renal pelvis that collects excreted urine.

Capillary Smallest blood vessel, with thin walls, across which oxygen and metabolic exchanges take place.

Cardiac Relates to the heart, the essential organ for the propulsion of blood to all parts of the body.

Chiasm The area of crossing of two or more separate pathways, e.g., the optic chiasm, in which the optic nerve fibers from one eye cross or decussate with the contralateral fibers of the other eye on their way to the brain.

Ciliary Pertaining to the delicate brushlike extensions on the free border of a cell that protect by propelling noxious surface matter from the cell. For example, eyelashes protect the eye; ciliary components of the eye suspend the lens and control accommodation.

Cortex Outer portion of an organ.

Deep Away from the skin surface.

Denervation The surgical, traumatic, or pathological stripping of the nerve supply of a structure or organ.

Diaphragm Muscular partition separating compartments, as thorax from abdomen (respiratory diaphragm) or pelvis from perineum (urogenital diaphragm).

Distal The portion of an organ or structure farthest away from the base point.

Endocrine Pertaining to glands of internal secretion, which have an effect on other glands or organs through hormones carried by the bloodstream.

Epithelium Cellular surface of the skin of the body, surface lining cells of the internal cavities, cells of glands, and important surface cells of the sense organs.

Erythrocyte Red blood cell.

Extension The act of straightening or opening out a limb.

Fascia The thin fibrous tissue that covers muscles.

Fetal Relative to the fetus, i.e., the baby in the uterus of its mother from the eighth week of gestation until delivery.

Flexion Bending or closing movement of a joint or spine.

Follicle Sac containing an individual hair shaft, a growing ovum, or portions of secretory or excretory glands.

Foramen An opening through bone or organs for passage of blood vessels, nerves, or blood.

Fundus The internal base of a globular organ, e.g., gallbladder, stomach, eye, urinary bladder, uterus, vagina, etc.

Gland A structure of an organ that secretes or excretes the product of that organ.

Glomerulus Nerve endings that resemble a tuft or cluster of fibrils; tuft of encapsulated blood vessels; the major filtration unit of the kidneys.

Glottis The vocal apparatus of the larynx.

Gustatory Denoting the sense of taste originating in the "taste buds" of the tongue.

Gyrus The elevated portion of the cerebral cortex (convolutions).

Haustra Sacculations of the large intestine (colon).

Hematopoiesis Formation of blood cells by the bone marrow, the spleen, and related lymph nodes.

Hemoglobin The component of the red blood cells (corpuscles) that carries oxygen.

Homeostasis The state of equilibrium in the living body with respect to function and composition of body fluids and tissues; the processes by which body equilibrium is maintained, e.g., temperature, heart rate, blood pressure, blood cell counts, blood sugar, etc.

Hormone Chemical compound secreted by the endocrine glands; internal secretions that depress, activate, or maintain tissue function.

Inguinal Relating to that portion of the anatomy near the groin.

Innervation The nerve supply of a structure or organ.

Integument The skin.

Intermediate Between two structures.

Involuntary (autonomic) Describing activity independent of conscious control.

Lentiform Shape of the lens of the eye or of the nucleus of the brain.

Leukocytes Group of six morphologic types of motile phagocytic cells in the circulating blood and bone marrow whose main function in the body is to provide a defense against "foreign" material (infectious agents, foreign bodies, abnormal proteins). They serve as reservoirs for many important effectors and mediators that are released following an immunologic reaction at the cell surface.

Levator Muscles having supportive and/or elevating characteristics.

Ligament A strong band of collagenous fibers that connect or support bones; also supports viscera.

Lingual Pertaining to the tongue.

Lipolysis Fat digestion and absorption.

Longus Long.

Lymph A watery fluid that may contain nutrition, chemical compounds, cellular elements, and waste products.

Lymphocyte A white blood cell.

Mammary Pertaining to the glandular portion of the breast; associated in the female with the reproductive system.

Meatus (pl., meatus) Opening of a channel of an organ.

Mediastinum Median dividing wall of the thoracic cavity, containing the heart and great vessels and the pericardium; separates the pleural spaces.

Medulla Central portion of an organ.

Menstruation Monthly physiologic bleeding from the uterus accompanied by the casting off of the cellular lining (endometrium) of the uterus. A new lining proliferates from the basal layer of the uterine wall.

Mesentery Thin membrane that supports the intestines and organs to the posterior abdominal or pelvic walls.

Micturition Act of urination.

Mucosa The lining membrane of the respiratory, alimentary, and genitourinary systems. This membrane secretes, excretes, and/or absorbs food and materials from the air and the glomerular filtrate.

Muscle A contractile organ of the body that effects movement and of which there are three types: cardiac; smooth, of blood vessels and the hollow organs of the digestive tract under involuntary control; and striated, of voluntary (controlled) muscle.

Obliteration Closing off of a vascular channel or communication, e.g., the cessation of blood flow in the umbilical vessels, ductus arteriosus, and foramen ovale after birth; removal of a portion of the anatomy by disease or by surgery.

Orifice Opening of a channel of an organ.

Osseous Relates to the bone.

Parietal Thin, membranous covering of the wall of a cavity, e.g., pleural, peritoneal; continuous with the visceral covering of the organs or structures.

Parturition Childbirth.

Pericardium The sac that provides the covering of the heart, consisting of a parietal layer and a visceral layer. The two form an envelope, with the visceral being the immediate covering of the heart and the parietal forming the external layer of the sac. Provides a smooth, movable surface within which the heart pulsates.

Perineum Area between the rectum and the symphysis pubis; the area through which the genitourinary structures pass.

Periosteum Membranous covering of bone.

Peripheral Away from the center: opposite of central.

Peristalsis Involuntary muscular contractile waves of a structure, which propel contents, as in the intestine, ureter, etc.

Peritoneum A thin covering of the interior of the abdominal cavity.

Pleura Thin covering of the lungs and thoracic cavity.

Pronation Turning the hand and arm so that the dorsal, or back, part of the extremity is in view from the anterior aspect of the body; lying on the stomach, with the dorsal or back portion of the body showing.

Proximal Point nearest a structure or organ.

Pulmonary Relates to the lungs, the essential organs of respiration.

Rami Small branches of a nerve or blood vessel.

Rugae The surface folds or ridges of the mucous membrane of a hollow organ. Distention of the organ flattens the rugae. The rugae greatly increase the absorptive and excretory capacity of the mucous membrane of an organ.

Serosa Thin covering of an organ.

Sinus A cavity or space lined with the epithelium or endothelium, e.g., paranasal air sinuses or blood sinuses of the dura mater of the brain.

Sphincter A thickened muscular band that controls the opening of a channel, e.g., the rectal sphincter.

Splanchnic Refers to the area containing the abdominal viscera; used to name structures passing into this space, e.g., splanchnic nerves, splanchnic blood vessels, etc.

Squamous Relates to the shape of one type of epithelial cell. Squamous cells are flat or platelike, as contrasted with cuboidal cells (cubelike) and columnar (columnlike) epithelial cells.

Stasis Stoppage or stagnation of the movement of intestinal contents, of urinary, lymph, or cerebrospinal fluid, or of blood due to disruption of peristaltic or pulsatory activity and/or by pressure from without by a disease process.

Subcutaneous Beneath the skin.

Sulcus One of the valleylike depressed areas between the convolutions of the cerebral cortex.

Superficial Describing the skin, or near the skin surface.

Supination Turning the hand and arm so that the ventral or palmar surface is in view from the anterior aspect of the body; lying on the back, with the anterior portion of the body showing.

Synapse Site of transmission of a nerve impulse from the axon of one cell to the dendrites of the next nerve cell. This site assures that the nerve impulse travels in only one direction.

Tendon The strong fibrous end of voluntary muscle, which is usually attached to bone

Tricuspid Having three cusps, or three points.

Trifurcate Having three branches.

Umbilicus The navel, site of the entrance of the umbilical cord, which contains two umbilical arteries and one umbilical vein during fetal life.

Vestibular Pertaining to postural equilibrium.

Viscera The organs of thorax, abdomen, and pelvis.

Visceral Thin membranous covering of an organ or structure within a cavity (e.g., pleural, peritoneal), continuous with the lining of the cavity (parietal).

Voluntary Relating to self-controlled, conscious activity.

Index

128

129